Avoid the Fate of Michael Jackson, Marilyn and Elvis

The Healing Power of

Sleep

"Avoid the fate of Michael Jackson, Marilyn and Elvis ~
The Healing Power of Sleep"

Century Wellness Publishing
521 Hammill Lane
Reno, NV 89511

Designed by Patty Atcheson-Melton, Wow Design Marketing, Inc.,
&
Margie Enlow, NuDirections Graphic Design Marketing

ISBN: 978-0-9848383-3-2

CONTENTS

Sleep

This book is dedicated to Michael Jackson, Marilyn Monroe, Elvis, Judy Garland, Heath Ledger and everyone else who has died or suffered serious health problems or drug addictions stemming from sleep problems.

FOREWORD

Medical professionals often mention some of life's greatest biological mysteries. Key among them include the inability to tickle yourself, the extreme difficulty in trying to sneeze and urinate at the same time, and the fact people often fail to smell their own breath.

Just as perplexing, many of the most puzzling mysteries often involve sleep, such as why we're unable to hear ourselves snore, why men often fall asleep within minutes after an orgasm, and the inability to recall many dreams unless actively trying to recall them immediately after awakening and the infectious nature of the yawn.

Dr. James W Forsythe's delightful book about sleep that follows takes a panoramic look at sleep, which not only expends one-third of our time on Earth, but also probably serves as the greatest therapy for the healing of a great many of life's health problems—including infections and serious diseases.

Any human being dying at the age of 90 has spent approximately 30 years "under the sheets," and not always in restful sleep. As Dr. Forsythe documents in this book, there are more than six dozen varieties of sleep disorders, some posing potentially fatal consequences. Anyone interested in this subject may already have some sort of sleep disorder, far from alone in this respect.

In fact, if you have a sleep disorder, your condition may serve as an indicator of an underlying condition in your body that may reflect a hormonal imbalance, or an underlying psychological challenge.

Added to these potential dangers, your condition might involve a mechanical airway problem involving the central nervous system, causing a common disorder known as obstructive sleep apnea or OSA. Loud and obnoxious snoring often accompanies this condition, considered the most common and serious sleep disorder.

Physicians know that obstructive sleep apnea afflicts one out of every five Americans older than age 50, while increasing in frequency due to the current nationwide obesity epidemic. Sadly, if left untreated, this condition raises the risk of heart disease, hypertension, stroke, diabetes and perhaps even vascular dementia.

Statistics show that more than 30 million men and women in the United States have struggled nightly with a chronic disorder that prevents them from achieving good quality sleep. Remember, the consequences of inadequate sleep, or sleep deprivation, has an impact on both our mental and physical well being.

Sure enough, the quality of sleep affects our personal relationships with our family members and our friends, as well as our job performance. More importantly, poor quality sleep might negatively impact our health and also lead to serious consequences, especially if performing dangerous tasks or driving while sleep-impaired.

One of the most striking quotations from the pages that follow comes from Shakespeare's "Hamlet:" "To sleep, perchance to dream." Surely much has been written about dreams in the psychological literture, especially observations or theories those posed by such great psychiatrists as Sigmund Freud and Carl Jung.

Some observers have concluded that the sexual content of dreams reaches its highest levels during the pre-pubescent period through the mid-40s, the point at which such occurrences experience a sharp drop.

Meantime, people afflicted by obsessive-compulsive disorders often experience recurrent dreams regarding phobias or travel. Just as distressing, some children who have seen scary movies, read frightening books or who hear horrifying stories experience sleep terror.

Deepening the mystery of sleep, both males and females sometimes report experiencing near-death experiences—the sensation of dying—after extremely serious illness or severe accidents.

Despite all these many disorders or challenges, throughout human history physicians such as Hippocrates and Galen have long appreciated and recognized the healing power of sleep. Today, many medical professionals know that ordering patients to rest in bed can accelerate the healing process, away from common stressors such as telephones, computers and family strife.

Unfortunately, however, when placed in a hospital bed many patients often get disturbed by the health-related procedures mandated and practiced by most medical facilities. These range from medical personnel taking vital signs in the middle of the night, to having to share a room with an extremely sick or obnoxious patient—possibly someone who snores loudly.

The neuroendocrine system heals our bodies during sleep, largely thanks to the production of vital hormones, especially HGH, DHEA and melatonin, secreted only during the deepest levels of the resting process. This, in large part, may be the reason why sleep—and especially high quality sleep—can be such a healing therapy.

Patients who suffer from Chronic Fatigue Immune Dysfunction Syndrome or fibromyalgia syndrome are prone to have poor-quality, interrupted sleep—and consequently produce very low levels of these important hormones.

Among men and women, the aging process causes increasing problems with insomnia and sleep deprivation. In women, this often occurs in the peri-menopausal years from ages 45-55, when the important sleep-promoting hormone progesterone falls sharply.

In males, the slow and progressive enlargement of the male prostate gland causes increasing nighttime urinary urgency, called "nocturia." This, in turn, disrupts high-quality sleep by forcing the individual to travel to the restroom every 2-4 hours on a regular basis.

Meantime, healthy people of all ages often experience a physiologic process often overlooked or taken for granted during sleep—the body's "detoxification excretory machinery." Many people are unaware that the kidneys often accelerate their filtration of toxins as the volume of urine increases during sleep. Also during this period, the colon keeps busy forming fecal material, eliminating toxins within the lower gastrointestinal tract, readying the bowel for early-morning elimination.

The complexity seems to increase, once we acknowledge the fact that hair growth accelerates during sleep, especially in unsightly areas such as the eyebrows, ears and nose. Many medical professionals believe that this signals the body's way of eliminating an increasing overload of potentially harmful toxins, especially when such buildup intensifies as we age.

Could it be that our hair is merely an excretory organ in many ways, designed by the body to eliminate toxins, particularly potentially harmful heavy metals?

Also, as we all know, besides the accumulation of mucous in our eyes and nose, we seem to sweat more during sleep as increasing amounts of skin flakes off—thus detoxifying the body by eliminating a host of bacterial, viral, fungal and heavy metal toxins.

Especially in the practice of Alternative Medicine, seasoned professionals know that people suffering from certain conditions such as the flu sometimes experience their worst symptoms during the wee hours of the morning when such illness often worsens—when the body's immune functions often reach their lowest levels.

Miraculously, during the later morning, the immune system rebounds and the body feels improved and certain flu-related symptoms such as sore throat, cough, headache and muscle aches often decrease.

For thousands of years, doctors have known that most deaths among seriously ill patients often occur from 3-6 in the morning, when immune function reaches its lowest levels—leaving the body less able to rally against potential death.

In laboratory experiments, physicians have discovered that sleep-deprived animals such as rats often become ill or unable to fight infection, leaving these animals unable to recover from what otherwise would be reversible illness.

With all these aspects in mind, just remember that "optimal health and physical vitality are just a good night's sleep away," and that the "healing power of sleep" is real and should be recognized by everyone interested in preventative medicine and self-healing.

Keeping this in mind, herein you're about the discover Forsythe's observations and answers to the many diverse, integral and mysterious puzzles that involve sleep.

How and where have people slept throughout history, and what has been the result of this evolution? On a more massive scale, you'll discover why and how younger people often can thrive on little sleep, while mature individuals often lack such attributes.

Pressing such questions further, we delve into a realm where people actually must fight or struggle for ideal settings or places to sleep amid horrific wartime conditions. Even in peacetime, as the years progress good-quality sleep often becomes elusive in many cultures worldwide.

As Forsythe points out in specific case-by-case detail, sleep problems or disorders impacting some of the world's most famous celebrities mirror difficulties suffered throughout much of society.

Causing even more concern, many tens of thousands of people die yearly in sleep-related incidents that you'll soon discover are preventable and often manageable.

Odd as this may sound, countless numbers of people throughout history have strived to deprive themselves of sleep with sometimes disastrous or harmful results—as you'll soon discover.

Adding fuel to the proverbial fire, you'll learn why people need or crave different durations of sleep at varying stages of life. All along, however, how does society discourage this necessary activity and what steps can you take to get necessary sleep despite sometimes negative feedback within our culture?

Learning what spiritual leaders throughout history have done to answer this dilemma should go a long way to putting you on the right and healthful course.

Amid these challenges, you'll also learn fun, easy-to-understand specifics on the biological mysteries of sleep. How and when do our bodies tell us to snooze? What happens to our organs and our body's cells while we sleep?

Just as important, at least from the perspective of maturing individuals, why and how can good, restful sleep potentially increase our life spans? Taking this a step further, you'll also learn how the body heals itself faster and with more efficiency while we sleep.

A sense of euphoria or at least extreme wonderment strikes some people, upon learning the so-called "miracle" of sleep—the ability of this activity to fight potential infection. How, specifically, does this happen?

And, on the negative side, how does our inability or difficulty sleeping promote or open the way for medical problems? Adding to the mystery, what causes each of the many dozens of sleep disorders, and how can we decrease the impacts?

Herein rests yet another puzzle, the pieces of which you'll soon learn how and when to put together. Specifically, what natural substances enable or promote our bodies to sleep? How can we safely obtain and use those substances to our benefit?

Among the most important lessons, you'll find specifics on why and how these natural substances decrease within our bodies—plus positive side affects that can occur as a result.

Just as important, what "non-natural" pharmaceutical products do physicians sometimes use to induce sleep for specific conditions? Far more important from the perspective of consumers, what are potential or common negative side affects of each drug? This, in turn, raises still another important question: "Why are sleep-related pharmaceuticals prevalent throughout society, and what potential harm is being done?"

As if all these many challenges weren't already enough, problem-snoring emerges as still another potentially serious health challenge. What causes this affliction? What can occur when snoring difficulties go untreated, and what solutions do physicians recommend?

You'll also find another clue to the mystery, the process of yawning—how that happens and why. Other signals to quality sleep include the rate and speed that you blink, the rate at which your eyelids flap throughout the day. Once you get these details, your perspective on this basic process is likely to change forever.

Many people find themselves in awe, almost breathless at least for a few moments when they first discover the intricacies of electrical energy that our brains emit during and after sleep. How does this affect your mental function and even your intelligence level?

You'll also discover specifics on the vital role that dreams play in our memories, diverse theories on why they occur and even some thoughts on why specific types of dreams happen—capped off by how these "stories" impact our emotional state.

Ultimately, you'll find advice from some of the world's leading health experts, who are increasingly concerned about the quality of sleep due to its vital role in the immune process.

Capping all this off, you also will benefit, discovering when and why it's essential to see your doctor for specific types of sleeping problems. To this end, you'll be given a pathway to establishing specific and predictable routines, designed to improve the duration and quality of your sleep.

Along the way, you'll be able to consider the risks and rewards of a wide variety of options, while realizing potential dangers and benefits.

Another important factor involves sleep difficulties among children, as you discover a variety of methods to identify and help alleviate such problems for them as well.

Perhaps most important, what positions should your body take while sleeping? Should you sleep on your left side, the right side, the stomach or back? How is each of these sleeping conditions likely to assist or accelerate healing of specific medical conditions?

The Healing Power of Sleep

Perhaps best of all, Forsythe shoots down the many myths and mysteries of sleep, enabling you to find and enjoy a personal pathway to eliminating stress, promote healing and perhaps even improve the overall quality of your life.

--Wayne Rollan Melton, Editor

CHAPTER 1
Sleep ~ The Natural Thriller

News flashed worldwide on the possible cause of mega-superstar Michael Jackson's death just five days after he died suddenly at age 50 in June 2009.

"This was a person who was seeking help, desperately, to get some sleep, to get some rest," Cherilyn Lee, a registered nurse and nutritional counselor who once worked for Jackson, told the Associated Press.

Officials revealed in the days that followed that police investigators found the powerful unconsciousness-inducing drug Diprivan®, generically known as Propofol, at Jackson's $100,000-a-month rented Los Angeles mansion.

According to various news media accounts, during the last few weeks of his life, Jackson complained to friends and medical professionals that he had not slept for more than a few hours over a period of days. Acquaintances told reporters that Jackson had begged them to get him the extremely dangerous drug, used to sedate or induce unconsciousness for medical procedures like surgery.

Lee told the AP that Jackson "wasn't looking to get high or feel good and sedated from drugs," but that the overwhelming urge to get some sleep motivated him to ask her for the drug. The AP also quoted Lee as saying she refused to get the drug for Jackson, and that she warned him of the danger.

Also to the AP, Lee recalled Jackson responding that, "No, my doctor said it's safe. It works quick and it's safe as long as somebody's here to monitor me and wake me up. It's going to be OK."

Even more disturbing, the media quoted Lee as saying she had overheard Jackson say: "Find me an anesthesiologist. I don't care how

19

much money they want...Find me an anesthesiologist to be with me here overnight and give me this IV."

Physicians and anesthesiologists later confirmed to the media that a doctor, nurse or other highly trained medical professional must be present when administering the drug—which can spark respiratory depression, resulting in cardiac arrest. The drug induces unconsciousness within seconds.

On July 4, 2009, three days before a scheduled public memorial service for Jackson, the TMZ.com celebrity Website reported that: "Michael Jackson made the rounds at L.A. doctors' offices, often getting anesthesia for minor outpatient procedures—procedures that did not require anesthesia."

In late 2011, Jackson's physician, Conrad Murray, M.D., was convicted of involuntary manslaughter for the entertainer's death.

The resulting media furor swelled into such controversy that on a Saturday, Independence Day of 2009, the American Society of Anesthesiologists issued a press release, stating that Diprivan®, or its generic name Propofol, is a "drug meant only for use in a medical setting by professionals trained in the provision of general anesthesia."

The organization stressed that the drug "should never be used outside of a controlled and monitored medical setting. Use of the drug should be directly supervised by a physician trained in anesthesia and qualified to provide physiologic rescue should too much drug be given."

At TheDailyBeast.com during the final days before Jackson's memorial service, Lee Siegel observed that "we are all hybrids to some degree, and fantasy is the only one of two places where our conflicting aspects work in harmony.

"The other place is sleep, into which fantasy sometimes rushes headlong when life overwhelms it," Siegel wrote. "That is the other, fatal, quality of hybrids. They hunger for—as the tabloids are putting it in Jackson's sad case—'potentially lethal sleep.'"

But why is the basic, innate human drive and desire to sleep so overwhelmingly powerful, so strong that an intelligent person such as Jackson would have taken such a huge risk?

Yes, people desperately crave and desire sleep, as instinctively as they want sex and food. For us, the nagging question remains, "Why does the body need deep rest, and how can we prevent ourselves from suffering the fate of Michael Jackson, Marilyn Monroe, Elvis and countless others whose lives spiraled out of control—largely due to sleep disorders?"

Sleeping with the stars!

Startled tourists from around the world did a sudden double-take, when they spotted internationally acclaimed movie star Nick Nolte, as he slept on the floor of a Hawaii airport terminal.

Curious fans and passersby snapped photos of Nolte as he slept in November 2007. Engine problems forced the delay of a commercial airlines flight the Academy Award®-nominated actor had been scheduled to take.

The news media and celebrity Web sites soon featured compelling images of Nolte sprawled across the terminal floor. According to some news accounts, the groggy actor born in 1941 awakened on occasion to chat with fans and to allow them to snap photos.

Just two months later in January 2008, widely acclaimed film actor Heath Ledger died from what a coroner described as a "toxic combination of prescription drugs," including sleeping pills.

According to some news reports, shortly before dying, Ledger started suffering from difficulty getting sleep and he tried to correct the problem by taking sleeping pills. A housekeeper found Ledger unconscious, naked on the floor beside a bed in his apartment in the

Manhattan community of SoHo. Emergency medical technicians pronounced Ledger dead at the residence less than one hour later.

A decade earlier in 1998, a newspaper reporter spotted Oscar®-winning actor Rod Steiger taking a nap on the Reno, Nev., movie set of the movie "Body and Soul."

"We need sleep to keep our sanity," Steiger later told the reporter during an interview. "Rest is good for the soul and for the body as well."

Steiger, who died from pneumonia and kidney failure in 2002 at age 77, had suffered from severe depression during an eight-year span, mostly during the early 1990s. Steiger blamed a lack of adequate sleep for some of his previous health problems.

Celebrities serve as an example

These widely acclaimed instances involving celebrities get mentioned here, largely because many people worldwide relate to such experiences. Tens of millions or perhaps even billions of everyday folks suffer similar problems, at least to varying degrees at some point in their lives.

So, what about you and the people you know? Have you suffered difficulties sleeping, or experienced excessive stress because of an inability to get adequate rest?

Just as important, what is adequate sleep? When and how should people get rest? How much snoozing is too much or too little? And what adverse impacts does a lack of sleep have on our lives?

At least during the young adult years from the early 20s to the mid-40s, the average person sleeps at least eight hours per night or a full third of every day.

At this rate, the average 75-year-old person has slept a whopping 25 years of his or her life. To this point, you've experienced the similar nature-mandated slowdowns on a regular daily basis—although perhaps without the consistency that you might like.

Whether out of habit or due to extreme sleepiness, for an extended period of each day, you've either successfully or unsuccessfully strived to get what some people casually describe as "shut-eye."

Yet, amazingly, most of us lack any inkling of what sleep does for our bodies. We fail to realize how this process happens. Our ignorance in this regard has become so extreme that most people fail to realize why we sleep at all.

What you fail to know can kill you

Did you know that without adequate sleep, you will die sooner than if you get proper rest on a regular basis?

Amazingly, our high schools and colleges offer courses on everything from mathematics to chemistry and cooking. But, sadly, our educational infrastructure lacks system-wide instruction on the importance of sleeping, how this process happens and what diseases adequate rest helps prevent.

When was the last time you heard of a college course entitled "Sleeping 101?" As laughable as this might sound, by having a far greater understanding of the sleep and resting process, you can position yourself for a healthier, more vibrant lifestyle.

From the start, the trick here remains to learn all essential basics of why we can and must sleep, in order to prosper and to thrive mentally and physically. Integral aspects of this mysterious process involve snoring, dreaming and even tossing or turning in our sleep.

Just as important, did you know that sleep enables us to grow throughout childhood, especially during the infancy and teen periods? Causing just as much concern, we lose many of the characteristics of youth as our sleep becomes less efficient from our 40s and beyond.

While discovering vital aspects of these integral life cycle phases, keep in mind that you still can discover new and vibrant ways to get adequate rest and sleep. Along this journey, many people find solutions or pathways pivotal in helping them to return to vibrant health.

CHAPTER 2
The merry-go-round of sleep problems

Oscar®-winning movie star Renée Zellweger, born in 1969, star of many films including "Bridget Jones Diary," "Chicago," and "Cold Mountain," once told "W Magazine" that her body sometimes fails to recognize when sleep becomes necessary.

Zellweger told the magazine that in the wake of a 10-country tour of a week and a half to promote a movie, at times her body failed to demand that she get sleep.

"But," she told the magazine, "you don't fight it, and you don't ask questions after a while. You just kind of let it happen to you."

Turning potential negatives into positives, actress, singer and producer Jennifer Lopez has been quoted as saying that getting eight hours sleep each night reigns as her number one beauty secret: "Sleep is my weapon. I try to get eight hours a night. I think what works best is sleep, water and a good cleanser."

Despite such positive actions, the inability to get adequate sleep continues to plague everyday unknown folks and celebrities as well. According to various media reports, in January 2008 "Grey's Anatomy" TV star Justin Chambers checked into a psychiatric ward to get help for a long-time sleeping problem.

"It's a biological sleep disorder," "People Magazine" quoted Chambers as saying. "Your mind keeps racing and your body is tired. It wants to go to sleep, but it can't."

Taking the need to sleep to an extreme

Unlike Chambers, who sought expert medical help in a controlled medical environment, some people seeking such assistance go to an extreme. Whether actor Heath Ledger knew of the dangers of certain sleeping pills remains a matter of debate.

The autopsy report for movie starlet Marilyn Monroe, found dead in her Brentwood, Calif., apartment in 1962 at age 36, listed the cause as "acute barbiturate poisoning." Some investigators attributed her mysterious death to depression, secondary to chronic insomnia.

While some rumors still persist that Monroe committed suicide, the possibility of a sleeping pill overdose also remains among possibilities often mentioned. So, was this sex goddess hooked on sleeping pills because of a problem getting rest or maybe even difficulties at relieving stress? How did Monroe face or acknowledge such an apparent dependency, if at all?

According to some accounts, rock 'n' roll legend Elvis Presley started taking sleeping pills in 1962 at age 27 to treat insomnia. Amid an apparent increase in these doses, did Presley progressively take steadily larger amounts of uppers and downers in order to persevere through each passing day?

By the time Presley died in 1977 at age 42 rumors had begun that he spent $1 million yearly on pharmaceuticals, including sleeping pills. Officially, coroners listed a heart attack as the cause of death. Even so, did Presley's initial insomnia problem eventually lead to his demise?

While these nagging questions pertaining to Monroe and Presley might never get resolved, your personal problems or challenges involving sleep today might have less or nearly equal severity. When learning more about the needs and benefits of sleep and of rest, you'll gradually perform a self-evaluation—perhaps in conjunction with a medical professional.

An essential first step often involves learning about the essentials of sleep and rest, before devising ways to benefit from these bodily functions in an efficient, natural and regenerative manner.

Consider our unnatural environment

While physicians and psychiatrists seem to agree that sleep in healthy individuals comes naturally, humans have devised stressful situations or environments that never existed thousands of years ago. These relatively new stress-giving conditions or factors involve everything from TVs and computers to cell phones, traffic jams and mega-crowded cities.

"Stress is nothing more than a socially acceptable form of mental illness," said Richard Carlson, author of the bestselling book "Don't Sweat the Small Stuff, and it's all Small Stuff." Carlson died of a pulmonary embolism in 2006 at age 45.

Although we might consider life's potential stress-givers as "all small stuff," some of the most harrowing environmental conditions we now face never existed just 100 years ago. Some medical professionals might argue that our minds and bodies never evolved fast enough to adapt to the many stresses caused by today's fast-paced technology developments.

For instance, Carlson died while on a commercial airline flight from San Francisco to New York amid touring to promote his best-selling book. Did the pulmonary artery leading to Carlson's heart sustain a fatal blood clot due to the stresses of traveling by air, rushing through airports to catch flights—situations considered impossible a mere 100 years ago?

In his groundbreaking book "The Naked Ape," first published in 1967—later updated and published in 1999 as "The Naked Ape: A Zoologist's Study of the Human Animal"—Desmond Morris describes the controversial qualities that people share with apes. If people still possess animal-like qualities necessary to survive, has our increasing technology and intelligence kept up with our basic natural needs such as sleep?

On one side of this controversy sits those of us who embrace Charles Darwin's theory of evolution or natural selection, believing that humans gradually evolved from apes. Others might argue in favor of Intelligent Design, which assumes our world resulted from an "intelligent cause."

Yet whatever theory or system people accept, there's little denying that thousands of years ago people never had to deal with the stresses of catching plane flights, having jets fly into buildings or the threat of nuclear attack.

Under this assumption, as individuals and as a society, we must develop and embrace natural, harmless and effective methods of getting adequate sleep or rest.

The battle for sleep intensified

During the height of World War II in the early 1940s, in London, England, and in Berlin, Germany, people huddled in bomb shelters or subways. Many individuals strived to get sleep as bombs dropped from aircraft destroyed much of the cities above them.

Throughout history, people have struggled to get sleep during harrowing or life-threatening situations, everywhere from battlefields to prisoner-of-war facilities to mass-extermination concentration camps. Condemned killers sometimes request a nap or rest time during the final hours before their executions.

While at face value such behavior might seem odd, through sleep and via rest nature provides soothing and healing qualities to our bodies and psyches. Undoubtedly, without getting at least some basic rest, more people would have died in concentration camps, prisons and battlefields.

An age-old proverb or saying has described consciousness as "that annoying time between naps." Some people have been known to joke that sleep is merely a form of caffeine deprivation.

Arthur Schopenhauer, a German philosopher who died in 1860 at age 72, seemed to put the vital and urgent need for rest into perspective when he proclaimed that: "Sleep is the interest we have to pay on the capital which is called in at death. And the higher the rate of interest and the more regularly it is paid, the further the rate of redemption is postponed."

Without question, as many medical professionals agree, sleep and rest reign as more than merely necessary. Each of these basic biological functions can provide the necessary regenerative factors, vital to expanding and improving the length and quality of our lives.

Put succinctly, "sleep is the golden chain that ties health and our bodies together," said Thomas Dekker, a prolific writer, pamphleteer and Elizabethan dramatist who died in 1632 at age 60.

CHAPTER 3

Great sleep can become elusive

For many of us, despite the natural qualities of sleep, good or nurturing rest often becomes elusive—while some people take such activities to the extreme.

"I've got to sleep 15 hours to sleep the way I want to," Mariah Carey, an actress and recording star born in 1970, told "Interview Magazine" in 2007. Such intense levels of sleeping far surpass the daily totals of 7-9 hours commonly recommended by medical professionals.

Taking her good-health efforts even further, Carey has been quoted by "V Magazine" as admitting that "literally, I'll have 20 humidifiers around my bed. Basically it's like sleeping in a steam room."

According to various news reports, Carey had suffered a temporary physical and emotional breakdown in 2001, when the star's Web site reported she had been overworked. Since 2004, Carey has enjoyed many professional successes, perhaps largely thanks to her healthy sleeping regimen.

However, even for people who strive just to get enough adequate rest to maintain good health, numerous sleep disorders can cause severe health problems.

At age 43, retired professional football legend Reginald Howard "Reggie" White, one of the National Football League's most honored players, died in 2004 after suffering from sleep apnea.

Potential severe or even fatal pauses in breathing can occur due to this condition, which some people believe may have contributed to White's death. A coroner listed the official cause as a cardiac arrhythmia or abnormal electrical activity in the heart, generated by a pulmonary and cardiac sarcoidosis, a multi-system disorder where symptoms include small inflammatory nodules.

Real-life tragedies such as White's death serve as reminders that when beginning to evaluate and determine your own sleep needs, pinpointing potential or existing health problems also becomes essential.

The stages of sleep also become critical

Kelly Brianne Clarkson, winner of the first season of TV's "American Idol" in 2002, once told "Self Magazine" that while she tries to start sleeping her mind begins creating songs and lyrics. According to news reports, whenever this happens Clarkson immediately jots down the information on a notepad.

"That's why I have a hard time sleeping," Clarkson told the magazine. "A lot of those times are at night."

The famed inventor Thomas Alva Edison, who died in 1931 at age 64, reportedly slept only up to five hours on some nights, partly in order to work and because he apparently considered sleep as an unessential waste of valuable time.

Others such as French sculptor and artist Louise Bourgeois, born in 1911, have striven to put the wee morning hours to good use by going to work during sleepless nights.

Embracing a sharply different philosophy, former British Prime Minister Winston Churchill, who died in 1965 at age 90, had been quoted by the "New York Times" as saying that by taking a nap, "you will be able to accomplish more. You get two days in one—well at least one and a half."

Some historians contend that Churchill claimed to have seen the ghost of President Abraham Lincoln while staying at the White House during World War II. Sleep experts may never know whether the famous nap-taker Churchill actually saw Lincoln or dreamt of the former commander-in-chief.

While some restless individuals might yearn to work or enjoy TV during any sleepless light-night hours, parenting commitments rob many of us of any chance to catch a snooze during the middle of the night.

"Everyone is healthy. No sleep though," Academy Award®-nominated film actor Brad Pitt told the media during the 2008 Toronto Film Festival. Pitt, born in 1963, and film star Angelina Jolie, born in 1975, have six children together, some of them adopted. "Sleep is something you long for, but it's all right. We'll get it."

Some people persevere without sleep

Perhaps eager for publicity or to gain widespread name recognition, numerous people have undergone significant feats in an effort to deprive themselves of sleep for long periods.

At age 17 in 1964, at least judging by some media accounts, Randy Gardner set a record for staying awake for a whopping 11 straight days or 264 hours—shattering the previous record by at least four hours. Numerous people since then claimed to have surpassed Gardner's record.

"I wanted to prove that bad things didn't happen if you went without sleep," Gardner said in a news conference shortly afterward. "I thought, 'I can break that record and don't think it would be a negative experience.'"

According to media reports, immediately after setting the no-sleep record, Gardner needed less than 24 hours to resume a normal eight-hour per day sleep pattern.

Some reports contend that in a rocking chair marathon, Maureen Weston of Cambridgeshire in England set a no-sleep record just seven hours short of 19 days.

In the Academy Award®-winning 1969 film "They Shoot Horses Don't They" starring Jane Fonda, her lead character, Gloria, competes in a Depression Era endurance dance that lasted several days.

Despite all these various claims and diverse historical accounts, some researchers contend that participants of no-sleep contests or similar events might have knowingly or unknowingly undergone intermittent periods of microsleep—the process of sleeping in spurts ranging from less than one second to 30 seconds. Medical experts say that even without sufficient warnings, such episodes can occur at almost any time.

"Sleep lingers all our lifetime about our eyes, as night hovers all day in the boughs of the fir-tree," said Ralph Waldo Emerson, a philosopher, poet and essayist who died in 1882 at age 78.

James W. Forsythe, M.D., H.M.D

Despite record feats, little sleep
can kill you

Despite these numerous record feats, nearly two out of every 10 drivers surveyed admit they have actually fallen asleep at the wheel. The surveys by the National Sleep Foundation also indicated that more than 100 million drivers, or about a half of American drivers, have driven during periods when they felt sleepy.

According to published reports, Richard L. Gelula, a foundation official, said we're "definitely on a collision course in this country" as increasing numbers of sleepy people decide to drive—apparently without "considering the inherent dangers they pose to themselves and others."

The survey concluded that 25 percent of people who reported that the quality of their sleep is fair or poor were likely to drive while sleepy. That compares to only 3-12 percent of people who enjoy good sleep, who indicate they would drive under similar conditions. Causing additional alarm, 59 percent of people who drove while sleepy decided to remain behind the wheel despite their drowsiness.

In its report, the foundation recommended numerous ways to prevent fall-asleep crashes, especially the need to "plan ahead and get plenty of sleep before hitting the road."

Motorists were urged to watch for warning signs that signal the start of sleep, such as heavy eyelids, frequent blinking, difficulty keeping the head up, drifting out of your lane, hitting rumble strips, frequent yawning, and suddenly trying to avoid a fall-asleep crash.

Sleep experts urge motorists unable to stop for an entire night to stop for 15- or 20-minute naps in well-lighted safe areas. According to the foundation's literature, caffeine and energy drinks take up to a half hour to enter the blood stream, and "blasting a radio, opening a window and similar 'tricks' to stay awake do not work."

Grim statistics for people who drive while sleepy

The National Sleep Foundation's report listed grim statistics for people who insist on driving although they feel drowsy. Among the findings reported by the organization:

• Annual sleep-related vehicle crashes: 100,000

• Annual sleep-related vehicle accident injuries: 71,000

• Annual sleep-related vehicle accident deaths: 1,550

• Annual monetary losses from such accidents: $12.5 billion

At these rates, each decade Americans sustain 1 million sleep-related accidents, resulting in 710,000 injuries and 15,500 deaths with $125 billion in monetary losses.

The findings also concluded that numerous other nations have much more comprehensive crash reporting systems, which more readily identify when sleepiness results in a crash. In those nations including Australia, England, Finland and other European countries, the report says, drowsiness contributed to 10-30 percent of all crashes.

Without question, the urgent biological need for people to sleep far surpasses the ability of many individuals to cope with stresses that might require or motivate them to drive.

The study concluded that people ages 18-29 posed the greatest danger to American society from driving while sleepy. Seventy-one percent of people within this age group are more likely to drive while drowsy, the report said. That compared to 52 percent of motorists ages 30-64, and 19 percent of drivers ages 65 and greater.

"There are compensations for growing older," said Cornelia Otis Skinner, an American actor and author who died in 1979 at age 78. "One is the realization that to be sporting isn't at all necessary. It is a great relief to reach this stage of wisdom."

Among other interesting findings, the report also found that overnight or late-night shift workers are more likely to drive while drowsy than their daytime counterparts.

"Sleep deprivation increases the risk of a sleep-related crash," the report said. "The less people sleep, the greater the risk."

CHAPTER 4

Some death-defying sleep depravation

As far back as the fourth and fifth centuries, some people have sat atop poles for extended periods of time despite the danger of falling asleep and then falling to their deaths.

Ancient literature claims that St. Simeon Stylites the Elder of Antioch—now Turkey—sat on a small platform atop a pole or pillar for a mind-boggling 36 years.

More than 1,500 years later, at least according to media reports, Daniel Baraniuk of Poland set the modern 196-day world record pole-sitting mark by sitting on a platform atop an 8-foot pole—while allotted short breaks every two hours.

Baraniuk's feat during the World Championship came eight decades after an American pole-sitting craze during the late 1920s. By some accounts, the fad began in 1924 when stuntman Alvin "Shipwreck" Kelly sat atop a flagpole for 13 hours and 13 minutes, after a friend dared him to perform the stunt.

During the next several years, at least judging from some reports, people nationwide surpassed Kelly's initial record—with one person reportedly staying atop a flagpole for a whopping 21 days. How could anyone have stayed in such a precarious position for so long, without falling asleep and plummeting to his death?

Apparently undaunted by such worries, Kelly became determined to recapture the flagpole-sitting record for himself. The media reported that in 1929 Kelly sat atop a flagpole in Atlantic City, New Jersey, for a mind-boggling 49 consecutive days.

Subsequent news reports claimed that the highly competitive Bill Penfield of Strawberry Point, Iowa, sat atop a flagpole for nearly 52 days, stopped only when a thunderstorm forced him down.

What about your sleep situation?

Of course, you'll never need to sleep atop a flagpole or stay awake non-stop for a few weeks, just to prove your own value to the world.

Still, these various examples have been given here to help drive home the point that people can survive and even thrive for extended periods without sleep.

For those experiencing current debilitating sleep problems, such heroic or perplexing tales serve as little comfort. People awakened night after night by persistent sleep problems often want quick or easy solutions to the problem.

Sure enough, nagging sleep difficulties can cause potentially cumbersome or harmful situations. Sleep experts tell us that poor-quality sleep causes inefficiency in the workplace, increases the likelihood of accidents, and even can result in severe mood swings.

Even more distressing, although certain individuals have clearly demonstrated that people can remain awake for extended periods, our bodies need and crave sleep in order to heal, to grow, to learn, to achieve or to maintain good health.

James W. Forsythe, M.D., H.M.D

Sleep essentials at any stage in life

Just as important as breathing and eating, sleep helps make life possible for all mammals through all ages of development—from infancy through the final stages of old age. This natural activity emerges as important for mammals, birds, reptiles and fish.

Especially in people, a lack of enough good sleep can cause a decrease in essential cognitive abilities, at least according to a study by the University of Pennsylvania School of Medicine.

"For sleep, one needs endless depths of blackness to sink into; daylight is too shallow, it will not cover one," said Anne Morrow Lindbergh, a widely acclaimed author and aviator who died in 2001 at age 94. She was married to American aviator Charles "Lucky Lindy" Lindbergh.

Lucky Lindy had gained sudden international fame on May 20-21, 1927, when he piloted an aircraft, The Spirit of Saint Louis, a full 33 _ hours in the first trans-Atlantic flight from Roosevelt Field in New York to Le Bourget near Paris, France. Besides striving to stay awake during this historic flight, Lucky Lindy battled icing, flew through dense fog, and used the stars for navigation when possible.

At least in part, the basic human need for sleep placed the pilot's son, Charles Augustus Lindbergh Jr., in a potentially vulnerable position. In 1932, an intruder abducted the 20-month-old boy from a crib in a second-story nursery of the Lindbergh's New Jersey home.

In 1935, a jury convicted a German immigrant carpenter, Bruno Richard Hauptmann, of first degree murder, extortion and kidnapping in the child's death and slaying. Hauptmann had 404 days or nights to sleep between the date he was sentenced and April 3, 1936, when he died in New Jersey State Prison's "Old Smokey" electric chair.

Yes, every story that involves people—whether their triumphant victories or shameful tragedies—involves sleep at least in some form. The integral question for each of us entails how we manage our sleep, whether we use the many benefits from this natural activity to our best advantage.

Sleep remains a mystery to researchers

The various integral aspects of sleep remain mysterious at least to some degree, according to scientists and medical professionals who have researched the many complex benefits and a wide variety of potential disorders involving this activity.

"The feeling of sleepiness when you are not in bed, and cannot get there, is the meanest feeling in the world," said Edgar Watson Howe, an American newspaper and magazine editor and novelist who died in 1937 at age 84.

Despite the many questions that persist about sleep, scientists insist that various studies prove the vital functions of this necessary function include physical growth, the relieving of stress or anxiety and the dynamic process of dreaming—while also serving vital roles in the healing or antiviral functions.

People who fail to get adequate sleep become more prone to mental disorders, disease, decreased efficiency in the workplace and perhaps even death much earlier than expected, at least according to many physicians.

"It appears that every man's insomnia is as different from his neighbors as are their daytime hopes and aspirations," said F. Scott Fitzgerald, a widely acclaimed American novelist and short story writer who died in 1940 at age 44.

During the months before Fitzgerald died, doctors had ordered him to get plenty of sleep, avoid strenuous activities and to rest after he suffered a heart attack while at a drug store.

At age 37, the day after his friend Fitzgerald succumbed from natural causes, an American satirist, screenwriter and author, Nathanael West, was killed in an auto accident in El Centro, Calif., with his new bride, Eileen McKenney.

By some accounts, the grief-stricken West, distraught by news of Fitzgerald's passing, ran a stop sign, resulting in the fatal accident. Would sleep or rest at home during that extremely stressful week have enabled West to relieve his mental anguish, thereby avoiding tragedy?

"Don't fight the pillow, but lay down your head, and kick every worriment out of the bed," said Edmund Vance Cooke, a poet who died in 1932 at age 66.

CHAPTER 5

Our society emphasizes activity rather than rest

Despite what physicians call irrefutable evidence of the urgent need for all of us to get adequate sleep, much of society imposes an unshakable stigma—mandating that we always behave in a high-energy state in order to achieve success.

A seemingly endless string of self-help books proclaim the supposed need for every individual to seize life in a proactive manner, constantly working to achieve goals.

Many parents and teachers urge teens and young adults to push themselves to their physical and mental limits, striving to generate seemingly around-the-clock study habits and to work as much as possible.

The 20th Century began as business experts and some philosophers embraced such comments as those by Jules Renard, a French author who died in 1910 at age 46: "Laziness is nothing more than the habit of resting before you get tired."

By the mid-1900s, the concept of getting much-needed sleep or rest seemed to get shifted to the wayside, as corporate America embraced the notion of "up the organization," a philosophy mandating that individuals should fully dedicate their lives to their jobs and to their employers—who, in turn, supposedly strived collectively to benefit society as a whole.

Even in the wake of the Great Depression of the 1930s and a severe financial downturn that began at the end of the first decade in this century, the overall news media conveyed the impression that life's most significant accomplishments involve work and employment. Upon clear observation of economic recessions, business professionals know that work and industry activities play essential roles in the world's financial health.

Compounding these stresses, in the social environment upon meeting new people most of us invariably ask new acquaintances that primary question: "What do you do for a living?" rather than focusing on health or environmental factors such as how someone feels or thinks about a particular issue. Instead of focusing merely on a person's job or work activities, would we contribute more to society by asking about matters of health and of the heart?

Follow the examples of spiritual leaders

A wide variety of spiritual beliefs or religions have stressed the urgent need for rest or relaxation, although much of society seems to ignore these necessities altogether.

History's greatest teachers ranging from Jesus to the Buddha and Mahatma Gandhi stressed the importance of adequate times for repose and spiritual reflection. In the Bible, the Book of Genesis tells us that God made the heavens, the earth and people during a six-day period, before resting on the seventh day—universally considered the Sabbath.

Bible scripture from the Book of Exodus says that one of the Ten Commandments that God gave to Moses on Mount Sinai essentially tells society to "remember the Sabbath and keep it holy," meaning in part that people should rest at least one day per week.

In Matthew's section of the Christian Bible's New Testament, Jesus stood on Mount Olive, weeping above Jerusalem and also visited there when Judas betrayed him, interrupted as his 12 disciples slept.

"Man should forget his anger before he lies down to sleep," said Gandhi, the famed spiritual leader assassinated in 1948 at age 78.

Through the ages, even agnostics and atheists skeptical of spiritual teachings have been told by scientists of the importance of getting adequate sleep.

"It is not the strongest of the species that survive, nor the most intelligent, but the one most responsive to change," said Charles Darwin, a controversial naturalist from Great Britain who died in 1882 at age 73.

Could such abilities to adapt or evolve in order to generate necessary change hinge largely on our natural skills at evolving and surviving crisis situations?

Perhaps inspired by either nature or by how society seems to tell us to feel, even where spiritual reasons seem unlikely, many Americans yearn to sleep—and they're willing to pay big bucks to drift off into dreamland.

In the United States alone, Americans spent a whopping $23.7 billion annually on sleep-related products—everything from mattresses to pillows, according to research publicized by the Marketdata Enterprises, Inc., a full service Florida-based market research and consulting company.

Americans yearn to catch a snooze

The "U.S. Sleep Market" report issued by Marketdata, examining the market and its components, covered everything from medications to sleep centers, according to information published by the National Sleep Foundation.

According to press releases or media stories, the report says that from 1987-2007, "Of a total population of 305 million Americans, 58 percent are estimated to experience insomnia symptoms or sleep disorders." Among other findings stated by these publications:

● Obesity: Consumer demand for sleep-related products has surged, as overall obesity climbs among the aging American population.

● Disorders: Increasing numbers of people tell pollsters or researchers that they're suffering from sleep disorders such as sleep apnea and restless legs syndrome.

● Stress factors: Worries of terrorism, longer work days and a challenging economy caused more people to suffer through sleepless nights.

By some accounts, since the first public "sleep laboratories" opened in the United States in 1977, from 3,500-4,000 such facilities began operations—conducting vital studies on the sleep patterns or habits of Americans, and also developing possible solutions.

According to information that Marketdata has printed about its report, this groundbreaking study forecasts the market while also discussing the "nature and structure, history and evolution" of sleep-related businesses.

In a three-night monitoring process sometimes costing $10,000, sleep laboratories use highly trained technicians and integral equipment check and record a patient's vital signs. These systems cover everything from EEG, EKG, pulse rates, respiration rates, oxygen monitoring and the timing or monitoring of restless leg movements.

U.S. presidents knew the important value of rest

Any sitting U.S. president gets hailed as the "most powerful living person in the world." Needless to say, great potential stresses and possible anxiety might result for these individuals as they make life-and-death decisions involving many millions of people.

So, well before modern polling and societal surveys that might have told them to seek out unique or restful environments, most of our nation's commanders-in-chief have made finding, maintaining and scheduling relaxing getaways a top priority.

Some presidents chose or created sparsely developed back-woods hideaways, while others focused on high-profile venues destined to grab the media spotlight. Thanks to intense media reports, some of these vacation sites generated widespread curiosity.

First Lady Edith Roosevelt, wife of Teddy Roosevelt, 26th president of the United States, chose two cottages at a 15-acre wooded retreat in Albemarle County, Virginia.

Although hailed as among our nation's most industrious presidents with many professions, Teddy had learned the importance of rest and relaxation after his first wife, Alice, and his mother, Mittie, died within 11 hours of each other in 1884—both of natural causes. Two years later he married Edith. They had five children together and also raised his daughter Alice, born two days before Teddy's first wife died.

Although apparently a hectic retreat for the Roosevelt's rambunctious children, the getaway proved restful for Teddy while he served as president from 1901-1909. The 36th president, Lyndon Baines Johnson, preferred to get away in the 1960s to his sprawling LBJ Ranch in Stonewall, Texas, especially as the Vietnam War intensified.

George H.W. Bush, the 41st president from 1989-1993, enjoyed vacationing in a Kennebunkport, Maine, home proclaimed as his family's "summer White House." He followed the 40th president, Ronald Reagan, who died in 2004 at age 93. With a much more laid-back style, Reagan vacationed with First Lady Nancy Reagan at their 688-acre Ranch of the Sky near Santa Barbara, Calif.

In 1942, as the 32nd president, Franklin Roosevelt became the first commander-in-chief to visit a former children's home at Catoctin Mountain Park in Maryland. The retreat became a favorite hideaway for every president since then, named Camp David by Dwight Eisenhower, the 34th president in the 1950s, in honor of his grandson.

While most Americans these days lack the resources or even the time to enjoy such unique getaways, the examples given by these and other presidents give the clear message that we all possess an urgent need for adequate repose whenever possible.

"Oh, sleep. Oh, sleep, nature's soft nurse," wrote William Shakespeare, the legendary English playwright who died in 1613 at about age 52.

James W. Forsythe, M.D., H.M.D

Skilled at enticing and magnetizing audiences from numerous social or economic levels, Shakespeare became a master at describing this natural activity, especially when proclaiming: "Sleep that knits up the reveled sleeve of care. The death of each day's life, sore labor's bath, balm of great minds, great nature's second course, chief nourisher in life's feast."

Cultures worldwide celebrate the importance of rest

Societies worldwide, especially those outside the United States, have for many hundreds of years or for countless generations celebrated a variety of diverse holidays or festivities—many of them focused on the importance of rest.

In fact, grammarians tell us that English-speaking cultures derived the word "holiday" from the words "holy" and "day." Many cultures consider the word holiday as synonymous with vacations and with specific days marking religious-inspired occasions that inspired vacations or rest.

As observances, many holidays in various cultures encourage or mandate rest and quiet time with ourselves, with friends or with relatives. Some cultures across Asia from Vietnam and Thailand to Cambodia and beyond stress the need to take a snooze.

In many cultures worldwide, Christmas Day hails as an official government holiday, even in cultures including the United States that lack or otherwise prohibit an official state religion.

Some economists insist the U.S. carries a reputation as the "wealthiest nation on earth," even amid tough economic times. Yet surveys consistently show that within a culture dominated by demanding corporations, American workers consistently complain that they lack adequate rest time or vacation periods.

CHAPTER 6

The corporate culture robs workers of vacation time

"Vacation deprivation in America is at an all-time high," Sally McKenzie, vice president and general manager of the Expedia.com, the world's leading online travel agency, said in a press release. "There are incredible health and wellness benefits associated with time off from work. Americans should take a cue from their foreign counterparts and relish the vacation that they earn."

According to an Expedia.com survey, the average American polled during the study period decided to avoid taking four available vacation days during a 1-year period. Could such motivation to stay at work result from stress, worries of a potential job loss—or perhaps even from a lack of funds necessary to enjoy a getaway?

For whatever the reason, according to the report one third of Americans "do not always take all of their vacation days." This happens despite the fact that one third of workers say that they feel better about their jobs and feel more productive upon returning from their vacations, the press release said.

In analyzing vacation habits among workers in Australia, Canada, Germany, the United States, Great Britain and France, the Expedia. com survey concluded that on average people in the U.S. received the lowest average vacation days per year at 14. That compared to: Australia, 17; Canada, 19; Great Britain, 24; Germany, 27; and France, 39.

According to some surveys, many people in other cultures are less likely than Americans to cancel, reschedule or delay vacations for work-related reasons. Meantime, polls such as the Expedia.com research showed that many people report they feel better after taking vacations.

During multiple years of surveys, Expedia.com said the United States has "the long-held distinction of being the country with the worst vacationing habits." This occurs although 52 percent of Americans who take vacations say they return "feeling rested and rejuvenated."

Rather than taking such findings to heart by extending their vacation times, Americans cut back on their vacations during the survey period—choosing to take one less vacation day than they had the year before.

The American corporate culture attacks the need to rest

Political lobbyists working on behalf of major U.S. corporations push against labor laws that might tend to provide what some people consider adequate vacation time for employees.

By some accounts, many U.S. workers receive only 10-20 paid annual vacation days, far less than their counterparts from Europe and other areas of the world.

Some labor unions and governments worldwide have increasingly recognized such disparity or vacation-related problems in recent years. In Japan, for instance, numerous holidays were moved to Mondays in order to give more people the opportunity to take short three-day getaways.

Other governments change such holidays in order to benefit the economy. Early this century, the Nevada Legislature changed the annual Silver State Admission Day or "Nevada Day" celebration to fall most often on the last Friday of each October rather than strictly on the 31st of that month each year—in order to provide a three-day weekend.

For most of the more than 6 billion people worldwide, life's natural and pervasive desire to get adequate rest and breaks from everyday routines motivates individuals to look forward to scheduled holidays. Our bodies require us to feel these intense emotions.

People sleep in coffin-like cubicles to catch shut-eye

Almost as if bumblebees returning to the hive, people in Japan have built hotels crammed with sleep cubicles—each just a bit larger than the inside of coffins.

The men-only Capsule Hotel in Tokyo's Shinjuku community charges about $30 for a bath and also rest time in a coffin-like cubicle equipped with a TV, radio, interior lights and a screen for privacy.

"What is the world coming to?" some perplexed observers might say. "Our world's overall population boom has gotten us to the point where people have started living like insects, or even as if temporary corpses for that matter."

Whatever the case, many people have begun accepting these facilities as a basic necessity for life. The need for sleep and to find restful space has gotten so severe that this hotel and several similar Tokyo lodgings even charge nightly fees to sleep in La-Z-Boy® chairs or recliners.

By some accounts, businessmen who lack time to return home for sleep prevail as the most prevalent customers. To accommodate such rush-and-go mentality, some capsule hotels enable visitors to brush their teeth or buy shirts, underclothes, ties and belts.

At up to 6 _ feet long, most sleep capsules seem large enough for individual visitors to get relatively comfortable. Numerous facilities sound morning wake-up calls, reminding visitors the time has arrived for them to jettison themselves from the cubicles.

According to numerous reports by the Japan news media, as the international economic crisis swelled early this century, many homeless young people began living at cheap 24-hour Internet cafes and in cubicle hotels.

Almost as if honey bees that communicate with each other via zipping their wings at certain speeds and manners, many of these people use their cell phones or by-the-hour rentals of Internet hookups to get on-the-spot, short-term, low-paying jobs.

Homeless people find creative places to sleep

Faced with limited options amid the natural requirement of sleep, homeless people across the United States have found or created many unique places to catch their winks.

Many individuals seek dry environments hidden from the elements, such as unlocked hotel lobbies, spaces under large trees, large parking garages or under benches.

Although this might sound like a cliché, the basic, instinctive need that all humans have motivates some of them to hunt for large, clean cardboard boxes for use as shelters.

For the homeless, much of this necessary hunt hinges on environmental factors, such as weather conditions, a region's overall climate and how police enforce vagrancy laws—if at all. Those without homes or jobs in temperate or coastal climates sometimes sleep on or near beaches. Other individuals feel a need to risk sleeping in public parks.

Taking matters to an extreme, in some large metropolitan areas many of the homeless sleep on stairwells, moving buses or subway trains. Perhaps most distressing, police say that many people intentionally get arrested on misdemeanor charges, just so that they can spend the night or limited periods in warm jail cells.

Worried that these people will take over entire public facilities such as parks, some municipal or country governments strive to tighten or enforce vagrancy laws.

"People who are homeless are not social inadequates. They are people without homes," said Sheila McKechnie, a Scottish consumer activist and housing campaigner who died in 2004 at age 55.

CHAPTER 7

The United States shuns the concept of siestas

Often even within or at least near work environments, many nations worldwide embrace and even insist on the vital need to take afternoon naps. Conversely, overall society and especially corporations within the United States often openly frown on such a notion.

Many cultures essentially shut down in the early or mid-afternoon, especially during naps that follow the mid-day meal.

Often referred to as "siestas," especially in certain Spanish-speaking countries, these periods of rest prevail in such diverse cultures, countries or regions as the Middle East, Spain, Portugal, Italy, Vietnam, China, North Africa, Bangladesh, Italy, Greece and Croatia.

Do Americans suffer from more health problems as a result of being denied siestas? And why does the U.S. culture scoff at the notion of afternoon naps, even at the workplace? Could corporate lobbyists play a negative role in this regard, failing to acknowledge studies that indicate productivity actually increases when people get adequate rest?

By some accounts, including information compiled by the U.S. Census Bureau, the small country of Andorra—sandwiched between Spain and France—consistently had the world's highest or second highest life expectancy at 83 years. Could siestas play a significant role in this tiny nation, also hailed as a tax haven?

By comparison, the United States ranked 30th from the top in life expectancy according to the "CIA World Factbook" compiled by the U.S. Central Intelligence Agency.

Countries much higher on the life expectancy list include nations where afternoon naps or siestas often are encouraged or part of the social norm, including the Chinese region nation of Macau—which often has the world's highest life expectancy at 84.33 years.

The many other siesta-oriented nations or regions with much higher life expectancies than the U.S. include Singapore, Hong Kong, Greece, Italy and Spain.

In 2007, the "Washington Post" listed results of a study indicating that people who napped in Greece had less risk of heart attack than in non-siesta countries like the United States.

America considers napping shameful

Americans seem to have considered napping as shameful since at least the early 1900s, more than one century after the initial Industrial Revolution.

The Protestant and Christian work ethics borne in Europe gradually solidified throughout most of the United States, especially after a massive influx of immigrants during the late 19th Century and early 20th Century.

Worsening matters, philosophers such as Elbert Hubbard, an author who died in 1915 at age 58, proclaimed such hogwash as: "The mintage of wisdom is to know that rest is rust, and that real life is in love, laughter and work."

Those considered genuine Americans emerged as people who possessed non-stop desire to work or to create and develop industrial machinery. Churches taught their flocks that slothfulness marked the plight of a sinner.

At least to some degree, these admonitions carried over into everyday life throughout much of America. Even through the Great Depression of the 1930s, amid massive unemployment people strived to work as much as possible.

To display laziness meant damnation in the eyes of many within the rigid confines of acceptable society, an apparent carryover from the Victorian era. Many people considered men who took naps as humorous buffoons.

These social mandates became evident in such sitcoms as "The Andy Griffith Show," such as a classic episode, "The Clubmen," which first aired in December 1961. That program starts off with gentlemen from a high-end men's club inviting small-town Sheriff Andy Taylor to visit their organization's club facility. At Griffith's suggestion, the club agrees to allow his deputy, Barney Fife, to accompany him there.

Shortly after getting the invitation, Griffith discovers Barney taking an afternoon nap in a back room at the sheriff's office. On the sly, the sheriff hides the deputy's shoes in a desk drawer amid plenty of canned laughter. Finally, after Barney's failed attempts to find the shoes, the sheriff pulls them from a drawer, showing them to the deputy—whose hair careens in seemingly every direction as if that of a clown.

After the deputy snatches the shoes and scrambles in a humorous effort to save face, Griffith smiles broadly while telling his deputy as the canned laughter intensifies: "Barney, I don't care if you take a little nap every once in awhile. I was just pickin' at ye."

Howling dogs prompt late-night anger

Social etiquette that frowns on the mere notion of taking naps fails to erase the natural requirement imposed on people by nature, the essential need for sleep.

"I'll shoot that dog if the darned thing keeps barking that way," some people have grumbled to their spouses, as their neighbors' animals howl during wee hours of the morning. Every night somewhere in America, 9-1-1 dispatchers get swamped by callers who complain of neighbors or party-goers who insist on disturbing the peace.

Noise pollution permeates much of society, especially in crowded urban areas, making sleep or significant rest difficult. Landscaping equipment, barking dogs and a maze of other noisemakers seem just as bothersome as commercial airliners, at least from the perspective of many people—left on edge by an inability to sleep.

Poor urban planning coupled with audio entertainment systems, massive street parties and the sirens of emergency vehicles can make sleep or basic rest a major challenge. Many physicians tell us that excessive, unwanted noise can harm our health.

Both on a physical and psychological level, excessive or unwanted noise can damage a person's perception of tranquility, a basic factor necessary for adequate sleep.

Scientists and medical professionals explain that while robbing us of valuable rest, noise can increase stress levels, make blood pressure surge, and create hearing loss or even tinnitus—a ringing in the ear that can lead to depression, panic attacks or forgetfulness.

Desperate for sleep despite their world-renowned work ethic, many Americans buy ear plugs or turn on huge indoor fans to create less bothersome "white noise" to block out much more bothersome sounds. Many frustrated people pack into city council, county commission or other government meetings to demand anti-noise regulations.

An age-old adage tells us that "you owe it to everyone—including yourself—to find pockets of tranquility in your busy world."

CHAPTER 8

Americans developed a creative resting system

Starting with the 1925 construction of the Motel Inn of San Luis Obispo at the Pacific Coast in California, on-the-go Americans developed a unique national system for travelers to rest.

The word "motel" first hit common dictionaries during World War II, a combination of the words "hotel" and "motor." Almost as if fast-growing cornstalks, motels shot up nationwide, especially during the 1950s as President Dwight Eisenhower created the nation's interstate highway system.

Americans increasingly needed places to sleep and to rest, as the widespread advent of the automobile started making travel easy for many Americans. Especially while traveling to and from wilderness areas, traveling motorists demanded convenient and affordable places to stay.

David "Dave" Barry, an American newspaper columnist and author born in 1947, has been quoted as saying that "camping is nature's way of promoting the motel business."

From expensive facilities to relatively cheap stop-and-go outlets, motels helped make getaways and rest possible to many motoring Americans—some for the first time in their lives. The earliest motels that spouted up along the nation's oldest highways such as the 2,448-mile U.S. Route 66, built in 1926 from Chicago to Los Angeles, became quick getaways—some facilities uniquely designed and considered landmarks within local communities.

Many of these post-war facilities featured unique characteristics, such as in the form of Native American wigwams in the Western U.S. to images or shapes that evoked perceptions of cowboys, spaceships or a wide variety of other marketing-oriented features.

U.S. Highway 40, which once traversed the entire nation from San Francisco to Baltimore, motivated entrepreneurs to build unique motels in a wide range of communities including Reno, Nev., Steamboat Springs, Colo., and many other towns.

Sadly, at least from the perspective of historians, many of these initial motels closed or sustained a severe drop-off in business when the Interstate Highway System emerged in the 1950s and 1960s. Gradually, huge corporations built cookie-cutter, non-unique motels near the new interstates, pushing many or most of their original competitors out of business along the older two-lane highways.

Ultimately, the necessary requirement that mandates sleep for all people helps the economy, forcing motorists to stop at least awhile in places that travelers might otherwise avoid.

Sleep motivated humans to create dwellings

Starting thousands of years ago, the very essence of sleep has motivated people to create adequate dwellings.

Unlike more ferocious mammals such as lions or hyenas that thrive in the outdoors, the more fragile human species developed shelters for individuals and their families. Almost as if bears or even rodents who dig out or find caves, people felt a need to put roofs over their heads—built from a variety of available resources ranging from clay, wood and steel to rocks, concrete and bricks.

President Abraham Lincoln proclaimed that "a house divided against itself cannot stand." Just as important, from the perspective of many individuals, a person without a reliable or consistent shelter often lacks the vital and necessary ability to sleep on a regular basis.

"What is more agreeable than one's home?" said Marcus Tullius Cicero, a Roman philosopher and statesman who lived during the first hundred years before Christ.

Determined to make dwellings the most restful places possible, starting thousands of years ago humans from a variety of cultures began creating various forms of beds. These entailed everything from mattresses and pillows to hammocks and stacks of blankets.

Instinctively, people knew or sensed that the more comfortable they made their beds, the greater their chances of achieving adequate sleep, relaxation and physical intimacy.

The age-old American proverb telling us that "you made your bed, now lie in it" drives home the point—whether intentionally or not—that the degree of comfort or efficiency of such sleeping places can play an integral role in our waking lives.

People often slept beside each other in a single room

Well into the 19th century, limited resources forced people across America to sleep in single rooms—sometimes beside people of the same gender.

Historians tell us that while a young man in his 20s, future President Abraham Lincoln shared a room and a bed for a four-year period with his friend,

Joshua Fry Speed. Following the customs of the times, through the decades at various hotels Lincoln slept on occasion beside numerous people, according to historian Douglas Wilson.

People in ranch houses across the nation at the time often shared beds, in some cases large families of at least five or more people. The practice continued to at least some degree in certain segments of the country, even as Victorian Era ethics or social conduct codes dictating strict moral behavior gradually spread across the United States.

In essence, people from various eras and social groups practice the acceptable behavior of their cultures to get their necessary levels of sleep or adequate rest. In keeping with customs of their era, Lincoln and Speed each married women; the Lincolns had four sons, and the Speeds had 11 children.

Healthy, non-sexual friendships and family bonds also sometimes grew as a result of the need to share beds for financial or logistical reasons. James Speed, an attorney and the older brother Joshua, served as Attorney General of the United States during the final five months of President Lincoln's administration.

Sharing beds to get required sleep prevailed as so acceptable, that numerous other cultures engaged in similar practices—which continue today in some areas of the world, primarily in regions plagued by extreme poverty such as various areas of India and Africa.

CHAPTER 9

Long-ago fables stressed our urgent need to sleep

Classic stories about the importance and quality of sleep spread worldwide, especially during the past 500 years as numerous cultures stressed the need for rest.

Hans Christian Andersen's classic "The Princess and the Pea," first issued in Denmark in 1835, got a negative reception from critics but became a favorite in cultures worldwide. The mother of a prince, a queen tests a young woman's claim of being a princess by placing a single pea at the bottom of 20 mattresses and a similar number of featherbeds.

The next morning this visitor, driven to the royal family's home by a rainstorm, complains that she has just suffered through a restless night—since something hard below had kept her awake, leaving an apparent bruise.

The gleeful prince marries this woman, after he celebrates upon hearing this complaint since only a real princess possesses such sensitivity. Despite negative comments from critics, many cultures embraced this classic tale as if innately knowing the importance of sleep.

"To sleep, perchance to dream—ah, there's the rub," said Shakespeare's Prince Hamlet in his famous and often-quoted "to be or not to be" soliloquy, written several hundred years earlier.

Indeed, audiences ranging from the lower echelons of society to the aristocracy knew the urgent essence of such statements—particularly when Hamlet lamented further upon the revelation that his father had been slain.

"To die, to sleep no more," said Hamlet, whose mother had married his uncle—the killer of the prince's father. "For in that sleep of death what dreams may come, when we have shuffled off this mortal coil, must give us pause."

To be sure, to varying degrees in a sense from the view of some people the nature of sleep mimics death, although only temporary as dictated by nature. Still, most cultures and the tales they generate embrace the essence of sleep as healing or short-term

Some tales associated sleep with evil

On the strength of numerous popular fairy tales or fables, many children embraced the fantasy that witches or evil queens imposed sleep on beautiful or innocent females as punishment or attempts at banishment.

In the eyes of many youngsters, sleep became both a permanent affliction almost tantamount to death, before ultimately emerging as a life-saving or almost spiritual condition.

Some observers might argue that these tales to varying degrees mirrored the general storyline of what happened to Jesus Christ, deep at sleep or dead for a period of time before a miraculous or spiritual awakening. Buddhists believe that 500 years before Christ, Siddh_ rtha Gautama rested, slept or meditated under a tree for 49 straight days before obtaining enlightenment at age 35.

To be sure, tales that involve sleep or awakening from apparent death grip the emotions among masses of people, instinctively aware of the urgent value of rest.

In the Book of John within the Holy Bible's New Testament, Jesus awakens Lazarus of Bethany from the dead, a condition perceived at least in the physical sense by some cultures as the ultimate, permanent sleep.

From the perspective of many cultures, a miracle occurs whenever we manage to awaken from death or on those rare occasions when sleep transforms our spirits for a greater cause.

In "Snow White," the German-inspired fairy tale that first gained widespread fame in the mid-1800s, an evil-minded queen discovers that a princess by that name hails as "the fairest of them all" throughout the land. The jealous queen recruits a hunter to stab Snow White to death in the woods, but there the man urges the girl to flee. Then, he takes the heart of a deer to the queen as proof that he had killed the princess.

Soon afterward, though, a mirror tells the queen that Snow White remains the "fairest of them all," living with dwarfs. Enraged, the queen makes two unsuccessful attempts to kill the girl, first with stay laces and then with a poisoned comb. But each time the dwarfs save Snow White.

The queen finally gets the beautiful princess to eat a poisoned apple before the dwarfs find Snow White in a super-deep sleep, unable to revive her. Assuming she had died, the dwarfs place her in a glass coffin. In original versions of this tale, a prince discovers the coffin and, magnetized by her enchanting beauty, he falls in love with the motionless Snow White still inside.

The prince convinces the dwarfs to let him have the coffin, which jerks or rattles when his servants try to carry it away. Snow White awakens when the motion forces the poisoned apple to dislodge from her mouth. The dwarfs help arrange a wedding after the prince proclaims his love for the princess. In romanticized animated versions, a kiss from the prince awakens Snow White.

Just as distressing, a wicked witch in the 1939 film version of L. Frank Baum's classic 1900 book "Wizard of Oz" uses poppies to put Dorothy and her friends, a tin man, a cowardly lion and a scarecrow, to sleep as they approach Emerald City. Snowflakes sent by a good witch subsequently awaken them.

In many ways these timeless tales and many other similarly compelling classic stories seem to mirror what our hearts and senses tell us about sleep, that adequate rest possesses restorative qualities that enable the body, heart, mind and spirit to conquer almost any difficulty life imposes.

Society makes the fairy tales come true

Myths and legends about the blessings of sleep have motivated people from many cultures to create shrines similar to those of the legendary Snow White.

Instead of mythical characters, however, these various tourist spots commemorate actual people from long ago, now on display as if deep at sleep rather than dead.

Claimed by some believers to have seen the Virgin Mary at Lourdes, France, in 1858, Saint Bernadette Soubirous remains on display in a glass coffin—a wax mask on her face and hands to make her appear as if asleep. Christians had unearthed Bernadette's body three times during a 16-year period from 1909-1925, concluding that her skin remained amazingly preserved. The Catholic Church canonized her as a saint in 1933.

A mortician embalmed the body of Argentina's beloved Maria Eva Durate de Perón on the night she died from cancer in 1952 at age 33. For the next two years, the corpse went on public display, made to appear as if merely asleep, a process some observers might equate to another real-life example of the Snow White process.

Following a 1955 overthrow of the government of Eva's husband, Juan Perón, the nation's new leaders absconded with her corpse, keeping it in an undisclosed location until 1971 when officials revealed they had buried her body in Milan, Italy.

Relatives later flew her remains back to Argentina, where they displayed the corpse beside the body of Juan Perón, who died in 1974 while serving as president a third time. With cooperation from the government, the family eventually buried her in a family tomb in a Buenos Aires cemetery.

Society's apparent yearning to immortalize the dead as if they remain asleep spans the globe, with both genders immortalized.

The Russian people put the body of Vladimir Ilyich Lenin, first head of the former Union of Soviet Socialist Republics, on display beginning shortly after his death in 1925 at age 53. Although this late leader's popularity has diminished somewhat in recent years, his body remains on display at Lenin's Mausoleum at Red Square in Moscow.

Russian authorities moved the body in 1941 before the advance of oncoming German Nazi troops, and the officials returned the corpse to the display site after World War II.

Of course, true, sound and nurturing sleep is for the living rather than the dead. Nonetheless, the fantasy brought about by images of slumber seems to put some people in a state of mental denial. Phrases that include the words "he sleeps" or "she sleeps" emboss gravestones within many vastly diverse cultures worldwide.

Popular U.S. film and TV star Joan Hackett, famous from the 1950s through her death in 1983 at age 49 from ovarian cancer, had often proclaimed her desire and preference for sleep. Good rest remained so important to her that humorously she ordered an inscription on her gravestone, still visible today at Hollywood Forever Cemetery in Los Angeles County: "Go Away—I'm asleep."

Rip van Winkle conjures up images of restorative sleep

The famed fictional story of Rip van Winkle, written by Washington Irving and first published in 1809, chronicles a man who goes to sleep for 20 years in New York's Catskill Mountains—before, during and after the American Revolutionary War.

Upon waking under the same tree where he first fell asleep, van Winkle discovers that many of his friends and his wife died while he slumbered. Before long various hen-pecked husbands in the same village wished they had undergone a similar fate.

Variations of the van Winkle story go back for thousands of years in numerous cultures, from Germany to China. Some fictional characters supposedly slept for up to 70 years or more, in some instances awakening wiser or with super-long gray beards.

Such fantasies involving sleep and the get-away from society that lengthy slumbers might provide crept into the film and literary cultures of the late 1900s.

Oscar®-winning actor Robert De Niro starred in "Awakenings," a 1990 film in which a medication seems to awaken patients who had been in deep states of sleep or comas for dozens of years.

Numerous science fiction movies featuring space exploration depict characters that go into states of sleep-like suspended animation for hundreds or even thousands of years.

Sir Terence "Terry" David John Pratchett, an English novelist born in 1948, has been quoted as saying that "fantasy is an exercise bicycle for the mind. It might not take you anywhere, but it tones up the muscles that can. Of course, I could be wrong."

Herein the dreams made possible by the sleep process, coupled with daytime or awake-time fantasies as well, bring forth a notion that sleep can enable us to escape life's many harrowing anxieties. Sure enough, as scientists and physicians tell us, the length and quality of sleep often play integral roles in assuring vibrant health.

CHAPTER 10

Modern technology improved the efficiency of sleep

From advances first made during the middle ages to modern technology, entrepreneurs have gone a long way in developing ideal conditions for rest and sleep.

Many long-ago cultures used straw for sleeping, while only the most privileged in societies such as the ancient Egyptians rested on beds made from metals, wood, stone or even gold. Historians say that some cultures even used old carved-out tree trunks for sleeping places.

Much of this became possible thanks to the earliest modern humans, who developed ways to raise mattresses above the ground to avoid pests and other potentially bothersome environmental hazards such as water runoff. Long before the waterbed fad of the 1970s and 1980s, more than 3,000 years before Christ the Persians filled goatskins with water to maximize comfort.

During the centuries before Christ, Romans developed mattresses stuffed with a wide variety of soft substances from feathers to hay. Many of today's bed manufacturers use the basics of these techniques. The early Romans stuffed numerous soft substances into bags made of cloth.

Many modern-day styles gradually came into play during the Renaissance about 1,500 years after Christ. Craftsmen used silks, brocades and velvets to cover mattresses. During the next few hundred years, the demand for adequate sleep motivated bed makers to improve and solidify frames.

The never-ending quest for superior sleeping furniture sprung to new heights in the mid-1800s when entrepreneurs patented and started manufacturing the first steel coil spring mattresses.

Thank a German inventor for your restful sleep

The next time you get a good night's sleep, you might need to give much of the thanks to a long-ago German inventor who died penniless.

Heinrich Westphal invented the innerspring mattress in 1871, but died without ever earning any profit from his unique creation featuring the basics of many mattresses that people enjoy today. Westphal's invention spread in popularity during the 1930s and 1940s, and ongoing improvements to all forms of mattresses continue to this day.

The Simmons®, Sealy®, Serta® and Spring Air® developments in the design and manufacture of mattresses by a variety of companies in the early 1900s helped pave the way for significant strides during the first generation of astronauts.

During the 1970s, the National Aeronautics and Space Administration, commonly known as NASA, developed a substance hailed as "memory foam." Made primarily from polyurethane and various chemicals, this dense foam naturally and immediately adapts to the shape and positioning of the human body.

The extreme high-pressure g-forces caused by certain levels of space flight motivated NASA scientists to create this foam. These developments soon caught the attention of medical professionals who sought to use the product for patients suffering from a variety of conditions, such as those bedridden from stroke and people suffering from gangrene, circulation problems or bedsores.

The specific needs of individual patients motivated researchers to develop various levels of firmness for "memory foam." In the early 1990s, Tempur-Pedic International, Inc., a major company traded on the New York Stock Exchange, developed a mattress comprised of the substance or product first created by NASA.

Consumers benefit from space-age technology

An independent company with international headquarters based in Lexington, Ky., Tempur-Pedic distributes products worldwide under the TEMPUR® brand name.

The company touts the technology first developed by NASA, hailing the product for its abilities to make the sleeping process pain-free— eliminating potentially painful pressure points, thereby decreasing an individual's need to toss and turn at night to find a restful position. Tempur-Pedic products range from mattresses to pillows.

This firm emerged as among a wide variety of businesses that tout themselves on the cutting-edge of providing sleep-related products—everything from beds, pillows and mattresses to pharmaceutical products such as sleep aids or medications for managing or eliminating the symptoms of sleep-related ailments.

Everything comes down to the fact that people need and crave the most natural, undisturbed sleep possible on a regular daily basis.

In order for us to understand the vital importance of this quest, many scientists, researchers and medical professionals first delve into the primary basics of sleep. From the start, this research involves getting a keen understanding of this natural process, why our bodies crave a restful state and what we can do to maximize these many benefits.

Could lengthy sleep enable our bodies to live forever?

Taking what many observers perceive as a futuristic leap, scientists continue to hone and refine the process of cryonics—preserving the bodies of animals and people in sleep-like states induced by extremely low temperatures.

Desperate to "sleep" within this state for hundreds or even thousands of years if necessary, some people pay big bucks to have their bodies frozen soon after death. Those willing to undergo this process plan to have their bodies revived from these frozen-sleep states after physicians develop cures for the ailments that killed those who were frozen.

According to some accounts, researchers have yet to develop a method of bringing mammals back to life after teams of cryopreservation experts first freeze those animals or humans. Complicating matters, current laws within the United States prohibit freezing people until after they die.

Experts in this developing technology stress the need to refrain from referring to the process as putting people in states of "suspended animation." Steady advancements in cryonics have lead to some public misconceptions.

From a scientific standpoint, while frozen the body and brain would lack the natural abilities to undergo the natural sleep processes, the process that would range from dreaming to rapid movement of the eyes. Nonetheless, the potential benefits made possible by cryonics motivate some individuals to seek benefits from its potential developments.

Legal disputes erupt amid controversial process

A legal dispute flared in July 2002 after baseball legend Ted Williams died of cardiac arrest in Florida at age 83. Williams' daughter Barbara Joyce Ferrell sued the late athlete's son, John-Henry Williams, who had sent the athlete's body to Scottsdale, Ariz., where the remains went to Alcor Life Extension Foundation.

According to some news accounts, as planned and in keeping with cryonics technology, professional technicians at Alcor separated the head from Ted Williams' body before putting the remains in a deep freeze reportedly almost 200 degrees below zero on the Celsius scale.

Amid the resulting controversy the news media reported that John-Henry's lawyer revealed details of a "family-pact" in which Ted, the son and the late baseball player's daughter, Claudia, agreed to be put "into biostasis after we die," giving them a possible chance for a future reunion.

Previously disinherited by her father, Ferrell dropped the lawsuit after lawyers for both sides agreed that a $645,000 trust fund left by Williams would be shared equally among the three adult children, at least according to news reports.

Could such disputes mark just the initial salvo of a massive legal war that might eventually erupt on many fronts? Whatever scientific terms experts might use for the process, the entire technology entails at least some form of "sleep," at least from the viewpoint of some observers.

For us individually and collectively as a society now, we need to concentrate on the basics that our bodies require today for good and adequate sleep—rather than solely focusing on possible future technologies that might not even prove effective.

Sadly, a vast majority of people from the very young to senior citizens lack any comprehensive knowledge of the basics that good sleep entails. Once we finish covering those vital and essential basics, great opportunities arise for ways to solve sleep problems that plague us today or to find, create or employ effective ways to get that rest.

CHAPTER 11

Discover the magical mysteries of sleep

Many scientists, physicians and medical professionals admit they fail to fully understand all the many mysteries of sleep. Even so, detailed medical research primarily through the last half of the 1900s gave an irrefutable conclusion about what many health experts now refer to as "a miracle."

Laboratory studies confirmed that the small pituitary gland at the base of the brain plays an instrumental role in the sleep process. Shortly after falling asleep, this organ performs a difficult-to-understand but natural magic show, pumping vital hormones into your body.

The process hinges on what physicians call the rapid-eye-movement or REM phase of sleep. About 20-25 percent of the time while asleep, your eyes move at an extraordinarily fast rate. Vital to keeping you alive, these episodes usually occur four or five times during an eight-hour sleep period.

Your body lacks the ability to heal without this integral process. In fact, you never would have grown in size, strength and mental aptitude from childhood beyond unless your eyes moved at this mega-rapid rate whenever you slept.

Your most vivid dreams occur during the rapid eye movement phase of sleep, a process some researchers believe plays a role in good or sound mental health. Under close observations in various studies, people deprived of the REM phase of sleep often suffer cognitive disorders or varying degrees of disorientation while awake.

Sleep enables vital hormones to enter your body

Primarily during the integral and complex REM phases of sleep, the pituitary gland deep within the brain shoots an essential hormone into your blood stream. These natural and necessary injections occur for very limited periods.

Medical professionals call this substance human growth hormone or HGH, which usually lasts in the bloodstream only for limited periods—often about one half hour at most.

Thanks to blood circulation, HGH courses into your liver, which uses this hormone to produce your body's vital and necessary insulin-like growth factor one or IGF-1 for short. A complex assortment of 79 amino acids form a chain that form this polypeptide protein hormone, without which you would have died during childhood.

Only as a result of IGF-1, your entire body grows at regulated rates beginning from the embryonic stage, through infancy and childhood. During the adult years, this same process proves integral and essential in the body's healing and restorative processes. Vital organs, muscles, bones and the skin depended on this hormone for you to remain alive.

Perhaps just as important, the body needs HGH and IGF-1 in order for wounds and significant injuries to heal. The body's natural healing powers never would work without this hormone, urgent for the healing of everything from broken bones to gunshot wounds.

Adding even more substance to the mix, physicians tell us that these hormones play a significant role in helping us maintain and achieve good health from infancy well into the mature years. As a result of these vital hormonal processes, the quality of life and overall health deteriorates for people who get insufficient sleep.

Sleep provides countless health benefits

Thanks largely to the body's essential hormonal production and distribution, virtually every function necessary to maintain sufficient or adequate health depends on us getting good, sound sleep.

Do you every wonder why doctors always seem to prescribe sleep, rest and drinking plenty of clear fluids as integral to curing practically everything that ails us? Have such statements evolved into merely clichés, something for physicians to tell their patients in everything from old TV westerns to modern-day medical clinics?

Without question, scientists and medical professionals have known of sleep's curing powers for many hundreds or perhaps thousands of years. Such prescriptions emerge as sound and solid advice to those of us who realize and respect the body's hormonal process. To think otherwise would be to deny one of nature's most integral commandments: "Get adequate sleep for good health, and in order to thrive in life."

Of course, only a certified, licensed physician or medical professional can legally recommend or prescribe sleep for any specific get-better regimen.

All along, many scientists insist that all of us should appreciate and practice good-sleep habits and lifestyles. To do otherwise would be to invite potentially severe health problems.

Pinpoint areas of the body that benefit from sleep

Whenever someone says things such as "hey, your skin looks great," you can thank the sleep process for playing a vital role in giving you such an aura.

Your personal libido, energy levels, the firmness of bones and the heart's efficiency all depend on the various hormones that sleep enables the body to receive, to generate, to distribute and to use. Even the memory, eyesight, hearing and levels of good cholesterol need you to sleep in order to thrive or remain at adequate or superior levels.

Especially from childhood through the young adult years, the quality and amounts of human growth hormone can increase muscle mass—while also helping to minimize the body's overall levels of unnecessary fats.

These qualities, in turn, often lead to the more vibrant and healthy appearances that many people enjoy through their young-adult years.

Partly for these reasons, physicians say, children through infancy and their toddler years and teenagers often need significant amounts of daily sleep.

Above all, at least when considering physical appearance, sleep can and often does help give us the appearance of good health. These factors hold true to the greatest degree into our early 30s.

After that phase of life, as the overall quality of sleep naturally deteriorates into our mature years, the trick to looking and feeling healthy hinges largely on our ability to get high-quality sleep at adequate amounts.

Our ability to heal deteriorates as sleep decreases

The body shows increasing signs of aging, as our natural production of human growth hormone decreases from our mid-20s to early 30s and beyond.

As we age, the pituitary gland steadily decreases the necessary amounts of HGH, and as a result the liver generates lower levels of the vital IGF-1 as well. Overall health steadily deteriorates amid weight gain from the early 40s through our mature years.

Homeopaths who practice natural medicine and even some standard allopathic physicians stress the importance of sleeping or resting as we reach middle age and senior status.

Even so, for most people the overall duration and quality of sleep naturally decreases at progressively worse stages in the 50s, 60s and beyond. This results in a proverbial domino affect, as bones deteriorate, heart efficiencies decrease, the skin wrinkles, body weight increases and the onset of diseases such as cancer increase.

A paradoxical situation emerges, when increasingly poor health often makes sleeping difficult for maturing people.

Nonetheless, good news emerges at least to varying degrees, since during maturity the body produces at least some growth hormones— although at significantly smaller amounts than through the young adult stage of life, when HGH levels often peak.

Thus, getting as much sleep as possible becomes just as important to seniors as for children and teens, except in a much different sense. At all stages of life, we need sleep for vastly similar reasons and due to minutely different factors as well.

Discover the power of rest

Largely in order to relieve anxiety and stress, our senses often command us to rest, a process closely related to sleep.

During rest or periods of relaxation, we strive to avoid any significant activities whatsoever both physically and mentally. According to some psychologists, sleep and its cousin rest can lessen or block anxieties or stresses that likely would cause health problems.

"Anatomy is destiny," said Sigmund Freud, the famed psychiatrist and master of psychoanalysis who died in 1939 at age 83.

All along, amid the ebb and flow of sleep and hormones that nature imposes upon us, each individual can take significant steps to make the most of sleep and rest.

"Adopting the right attitude can convert a negative stress into a positive one," said Hans Hugo Bruno Selye, a Canadian endocrinologist who died in 1982 at age 75.

Besides consciously taking positive action, we also can listen and respond to what our hearts, bodies and senses tell us about the need to rest or sleep at any given time. For this to happen, you need to set aside some potentially stressful demands imposed by today's round-the-clock, do-everything society.

Lilly Tomlin, an American comedienne born in 1939, has been quoted as saying that "for fast-acting relief try slowing down."

Especially for middle-aged people and seniors, the trick here involves recognizing the need for physical and mental down time—and taking necessary action to make that happen. Anyone who often complains or mumbles that "I need a rest" should seize the moment and do just that.

How often have you heard of instances where people have worked for many decades at a job before finally retiring, only to die of a heart attack or stroke within mere weeks or months after finally pulling the cords on their golden parachutes? Could an inability or difficulty to relax play a negative role in at least some of these tragic situations?

"Brain cells create ideas; stress kills brain cells," wrote Richard Saunders, the pseudonym of Benjamin Franklin, an American founding father and statesman who died in 1790 at age 84. "Stress is not a good idea."

Recognize these twin culprits

Some psychology and mental health experts actually claim that stress and anxiety hail as mere products of our minds, rather than actual physical conditions.

One widely acclaimed popular American self-help advocate, unworthy of being named here, has even gone so far as to insist that "the components of anxiety, stress, fear and anger do not exist independently of you in the world. They simply do not exist in the physical world, even though we talk about them as if they do."

Such nonsense flies in the face of renowned experts who know that to say stress and anxiety never existed would be like throwing manure at a high-power electric fan. The mess could very well fly back straight at such malcontents.

Today's mental institutions host countless numbers of people plagued by fear and excessive worry. Physicians prescribe hundreds of billions of dollars yearly in anti-depressant and anti-stress pharmaceuticals. Anxiety sometimes results from threats or risk factors, either real or perceived.

Compounding these problems, a failure to get adequate sleep can result in anxious or stress-filled behavior marked by fits of anger or rage, according to some health experts.

In medical terms, stress occurs when the body fails to respond either physically or emotionally to various dangers, whether real or perceived.

Some people suffering from stress undergo symptoms similar to those experienced by individuals who fail to get adequate sleep. Physicians tell us that besides headaches and racing hearts, those suffering from severe stress often become irritable or face extreme difficulties when trying to concentrate.

Andrew Denton, an Australian comic born in 1960, has been quoted as saying that "pressure and stress is the common cold of the psyche."

Whether such observations seem valid comes as little consolation to some people who fail to get adequate sleep or rest, possibly suffering from severe stress as a result.

In 1995, "People Magazine" quoted American business magnate Martha Stewart as saying that she slept only four hours each night. Seven years later in 2002, CBS-TV anchor Jane Clayson asked Stewart about legal problems that the businesswoman faced at the time regarding alleged improprieties in stock transactions.

"I just want to focus on my salad," Stewart said in a response that soon gained widespread notoriety.

Would this widely admired billionaire have given a more direct and concise response, had she been able or willing to sleep more at night? Is it possible that insufficient sleep played a negative role in Stewart's personal problems, which lead to a 2004 conviction of conspiracy, obstruction and making false statements to investigators?

Answers to such queries might never come forth. Nonetheless, countless situations involving other individuals lead us to conclude that insufficient sleep or rest can and does play a negative role in contributing to unnecessary stress—and negative behaviors that can occur as a result.

Outside factors cause stress and sleep problems

Factors outside our control often cause stressful situations that rob us of the ability to sleep—which, ironically, helps play a key role in enabling us to relieve stress.

Following allegations that he showed up drunk at a 2009 press conference, Shoichi Nakagawa resigned as Japan's finance minister.

Denying any problem with alcohol, Nakagawa blamed sleep problems caused by the combination of jet leg and medications.

In a 1964 episode of the hit NBC-TV western "Bonanza," the character Little Joe played by the late actor Michael Landon, tosses and turns at night—unable to sleep, plagued by nightmares about his fear of heights. Little Joe's lack of sleep made him stressful, snipping and speaking harshly to relatives. This young man's severe anxiety finally tapers off, after his father Ben Cartwright tricks him to climb a high ridge, proving that Little Joe could overcome fear.

For thousands of years, people from many diverse cultures have equated sleep with darkness and even death, despite the important healing powers of such activity.

In Greek Mythology, Hypnos personified sleep, while his twin Thanatos represented death and their mother, the goddess Nyx, signified the essence of "night." Hypnos resided in a dark cave, apparently to signify the period when most people sleep—before and after sundown.

Some observers might argue that in a sense Hypnos helps relieve stress for Endymion, sentenced by Zeus to eternal sleep. Hypnos empowers Endymion to sleep with his eyes open. This, in turn, enables Endymion to always watch his beloved Selene, goddess of the moon.

Tales such as these signify that perhaps ancient cultures realized that variations of light and dark play significant roles in when and how we sleep. Without such a light-and-dark process, sleep problems may result, causing stress and wreaking havoc upon our lives.

CHAPTER 12

Melatonin serves a vital role in your sleep

In nature, people find themselves naturally inclined to stay awake for the most part during daylight hours, while more likely to sleep when dark prevails.

A natural substance within the body makes this possible. When a new day's light first streams into your sleeping quarters, melatonin pulsating through the body senses this change and prompts you to awaken—at least during healthy conditions.

The small pineal gland within the brain produces this vital substance. Like the pituitary gland that produces growth hormone, which also sits in the brain, the pineal gland serves an essential role in or during the sleep process.

The pineal gland contains at least 100 times more serotonin than any other area of the body. This proves significant because while serving as an important communicator within the central nervous system, serotonin—a direct precursor of melatonin—helps the body regulate a wide range of vital functions including sleep, sexuality and metabolism.

From the perspective of physicians, serotonin serves as a thermostat when working in conjunction with the distribution of HGH, the pituitary and the hypothalamus—which sits in the brain above the pituitary gland.

Think of this as sort of a thermostat system in your home, which essentially shuts off the heater or air conditioner when certain pre-designated temperatures emerge. Your body's regulation system shuts on melatonin or serotonin production when HGH production reaches maximum levels.

Under normal and regular conditions, the body senses when to make such changes kick into gear. But within an individual person these internal systems can fall off the structured pattern due to activities such as modern jet flight—when travelers suddenly find themselves in different time zones. Such quick swings between vastly different phases of dark or light conditions can result in what many travelers call "jet lag."

Melatonin performs many other benefits

Determined to battle the negative affects of jet lag, including disturbed sleep patterns and inconsistent appetites, some seasoned travelers recommend using melatonin—a natural, non-steroidal hormone.

Although this substance naturally produced within the body also is available over-the-counter at pharmacies or grocery stores, women trying to conceive or those already pregnant or nursing, should avoid such products. Besides regulating sleep periods, among the many benefits or findings that physicians say melatonin provides:

• Life spans: At least in Russian studies, melatonin extended the life spans of mice by 25 percent.

• Eliminate toxins: Melatonin battles free radicals that can accelerate the aging process, generated from contaminated water, food and the environment.

● Prevents cancer: This natural substance also wards off or fights cancers, according to studies at the University of Texas Health Center at San Antonio.

● Prevents osteoporosis: As an essential hormone, melatonin fends off the weakening of the bones, of concern to maturing people—especially women.

Also, people can learn to take better advantage of the melatonin that their bodies already produce. For instance, an individual who finds getting up in the mornings difficult might try to leave curtains open, enabling the body's natural melatonin the kick into gear.

Meantime, some people who work graveyard or swing shifts and who sleep much or almost all of available daylight hours, might consider taking melatonin pills—while also keeping their bedrooms or sleeping areas as dark as possible during their sleep periods.

"There is never time in the future in which we will work out our salvation," said James Arthur Baldwin, an American writer, novelist and social activist who died in 1987 at age 63. "The challenge is in the moment; the time is always now."

The aging process decreases melatonin production

While the body's production of growth hormone lessens as we age, the body's natural production and effectiveness of melatonin goes haywire as a result.

At about age 70, melatonin levels have decreased to 15-20 percent of their range during youth, far below their peak levels from our mid-teens to mid-20s.

These life-cycle changes in the body's hormonal process make sleep increasingly difficult or seeming less urgent for maturing people. This destructive cyclone contributes to worsening health since the body need HGH and melatonin to battle or prevent certain diseases and signs of advanced years.

"These are the soul's changes," said Virginia Woolf, a British essayist and novelist who died in 1941 at age 59. "I don't believe in aging. I believe in forever altering one's aspect of the sun. Hence my optimism."

Realizing the body's decrease in HGH and melatonin during maturity, homeopaths and other medical professionals stress the importance of getting as much sleep as reasonably possible during life's senior phase.

"I could not, at any age, be content to make my place in a corner by the fireside and simply look on," said former First Lady Eleanor Roosevelt, who died in 1962 at age 78.

Amid today's can-do, keep-vibrant society that urges seniors to remain active, people within this life phase still need to embrace the importance of rest and good sleep. All along, seniors still could pursue or enjoy vibrant activities, important to a full and zestful life during any age.

"The secret of genius is to carry the spirit of the child into old age, which means never losing your enthusiasm," said Aldous Leonard Huxley, an English writer who died in 1963 at age 69.

James W. Forsythe, M.D., H.M.D

Decreased melatonin levels
harm the body

The body's significant decreases in melatonin among mature people can generate negative or harmful conditions, including depression or even sleep apnea—a potentially fatal condition.

A severe disorder, sleep apnea causes life-threatening conditions, intermittent periods when people stop breathing at stretches of 30 seconds or more while asleep. Sometimes breathing fails to resume, resulting in death.

Sadly, many people who suffer from sleep apnea never realize the condition endangers them. According to various published reports, an individual who undergoes at least five stop-breathing episodes per hour during sleep suffers from clinically significant levels of sleep apnea. People with sleep apnea also complain of suffering from fatigue or sleepiness during non-sleep periods of the day.

According to some physicians and various medical reports, numerous people with severe cases of the obstructive form of sleep apnea also suffer from:

● **Congestive heart failure**: In this often deadly condition, the heart lacks the ability to keep the blood flowing at levels necessary for good health.

● **Hypercapnia**: Carbon dioxide builds within the body to extremely dangerous levels, potentially resulting in high blood pressure, panic attacks or even death.

● **Hypoxemia**: The body gets insufficient oxygen levels, abnormally low amounts within the blood supply.

- **Sleep deprivation**: A person who fails to get adequate amounts of sleep might suffer from a wide variety of negative conditions, including constipation, daytime drowsiness, irritability, weakened immune systems and many other adverse symptoms.

- **Other symptoms**: According to a variety of news reports or professional medical articles, other potentially significant symptoms include diabetes, stroke, high blood pressure and cardiovascular disease.

Worsening matters, obese people or individuals who recently gained lots of weight might become more prone to sleep apnea, at least according to some studies. From the perspective of individuals who stay in the same rooms as people who have sleep apnea, the condition sometimes becomes disruptive.

Published reports indicate that some physicians seek to treat obstructive forms of sleep apnea by encouraging such individuals to lose weight, stop smoking or avoid certain substances such as alcohol or pharmaceutical products that relax the muscles.

An American Journal of Respiratory and Clinical Care Medicine report said that some sleep apnea suffers benefit if they snooze with their upper bodies elevated by at least 30 degrees. For complex forms of sleep apnea, numerous dentists use Oral Appliance Therapy, inserting custom-made mouthpieces to open airways.

The National Heart, Blood and Lung Institute has used Continuous Positive Airway Pressure or CPAP machines to gently blow air into the throats of people who suffer from sleep apnea.

CHAPTER 13

Numerous deadly sleep-related afflictions

Numerous harmful medical conditions can occur during sleep, despite the tremendous overall health benefits such activity provides.

Sudden infant death syndrome, sometimes called SIDS, has emerged among the most feared and dreaded sleep disorders. By some accounts, about one out of every 2,000 births in the United States results in an infant who dies suddenly and without warning while sleeping.

According to an article from Scripts Howard News Service, 2,247 infants died from SIDS in the U.S. in 2004, down from 4,895 such fatalities during 1992.

Sadly, scientists, physicians and medical professionals admit they still need to determine a specific cause for this heart-breaking syndrome. An age-old saying tells us that when we die, "all that we have is left to others; all that we are we take with us."

Infants who pass away from this syndrome, typically between one month and one year old, leave us, with their potential unfulfilled — taking with them the hope and promise of long and exploring lives.

While experts lack specific, undisputable causes for SIDS, suspected potential culprits have ranged from brain stem abnormalities to bacteria or staph infections.

Perhaps precautions against SIDS might help

Although medical experts still strive to determine specific or irre-futable causes for sudden infant death syndrome, some precautions have been recommended or suggested by various individual physi-cians or health-related institutions. Among them:

● **Prone position**: The American Journal of Public Health dis-cussed recommendations that infants sleep on their backs or sides, rather than stomachs. Meantime, a study by some researchers indi-cated that infants who sleep on their tummies develop superior mo-tor skills and social skills than babies who sleep on their backs.

● **Mother's health**: Various researchers reportedly believe that women who fail to care for their own health while pregnant might increase their child's risk of SIDS. Specific documentation on this claim seems sparse or nil, although physicians recommend that all pregnant women concentrate on optimal pre-natal care.

● **Teen pregnancies**: The American Sudden Infant Death Syndrome Institute has indicated that babies produced by teenage girls might have a greater incidence of SIDS. Among various recommendations published or publicized by the institute:

● **Frequency**: Avoid having multiple pregnancies during one-year periods.

● **Drugs**: Avoid heroin, smoking or tobacco while pregnant.

● **Rooms**: Have the baby sleep in the parent's room until at least six months old.

● **Beds**: Put babies on firm mattresses in beds designed for infants.

● **Solitude**: Avoid placing anything other than the baby in the infant's bed, which should never contain toys, covers, bumper pads, positioning devices or pillows.

● **Placement**: Always put infants in their own beds, and never in adult beds, which experts consider unsafe for babies.

● **Environment**: Set room temperatures at levels that adults consider comfortable. Put enough clothes on the infant to make the little person comfortable and warm, yet avoid putting too much clothing on the child.

● **Adults**: Partly to avoid rolling over and inadvertently smothering an infant, never sleep on an adult bed or a couch with the child.

● **Pacifiers**: Some studies indicate a lower instance of SIDS among infants who use pacifiers. So, consider offering such devices to your baby.

● **Avoidance**: Keep the child away from people who have been exposed to infections, tobacco, crowds, and individuals with unwashed hands.

● **Meals**: Whenever possible, breastfeed the infant, since doing so can decrease the likelihood of certain digestive or breathing infections.

● **Cleanliness**: Keep everything clean that the baby gets close to or touches.

● **Care givers**: Tell anyone assigned to care for the child to take these precautions.

The Institute and physicians urge parents or care givers to contact a doctor right away if the infant suffers various medical conditions. Adverse symptoms might range from turning blue or stops in breathing to gagging or spitting up.

"Trust yourself. You know more than you think you do," said Dr. Benjamin Spock, a famed pediatrician and author of "Baby and Child Care," who died in 1998 at age 94.

"The more people have studied what is best for children, the more they have come to the conclusion that what good mothers and fathers instinctively feel like doing for their babies is best after all," said Spock, an expert at psychoanalyzing the interactions of infants and family members.

Snoring involves a natural process

Seemingly almost everyone from princes to paupers snores on occasion, as dictated by the biological makeup of the human condition.

By some accounts, the late former British Prime Minister Winston Churchill snored often, especially after excessive cigar smoking and alcohol consumption. Theodore "Teddy" Roosevelt, 26th president of the United States, was only 60 years old when he died in his sleep in 1919, from an apparent coronary embolism and an apparent 2 _ –month bout of rheumatism—marked by excessive snoring.

According to some reports, his cousin Franklin Delano Roosevelt, the 32nd President of the United States who died in 1945 at age 63, suffered from sleep apnea.

The United Kingdom's Queen Victoria, who died of a stroke in 1901 at age 81, reportedly developed a very loud snoring condition as her weight ballooned as she aged.

The snoring problems of the extremely rich and mega-famous mirror those of countless common people worldwide, seemingly throughout recorded history.

According to a story distributed by BBC News, 40 percent of middle-aged people snore, mirroring the percentage of women who snore—while half of men experience this condition. Altough such statistics seem to vary depending on specific studies involved, overall conclusions proclaim that many people snore.

Technically, snoring occurs when obstructions block or hinder the natural air flow in the breathing process, thereby creating sound that can become soft or even annoyingly loud. Some studies indicate the propensity of numerous people to snore increases as they mature, particularly past age 60.

Various other potential or possible causes include nasal passage obstructions, throat muscles that become too weak, weight gain that results in more fat near or within the throat, and tensions that cause muscles within the jaw to become misaligned.

Snoring symptoms can become serious

Snoring can cause a wide variety of extensive health problems, according to the "Journal of Clinical Endocrinology & Metabolism."

Ultimately, snoring can cause sleep deprivation where the most severe symptoms include extreme mental depression. Besides decreases in sex drives, people who snore also might become irritable, experience difficulty concentrating and become excessively drowsy during periods when they want to remain awake.

Worsening matters, as reported by the BBC, some sleep experts and researchers believe that snorers may face a greater risk of heart attack than non-snorers.

An article distributed by the Associated Professional Sleep Societies indicates a greater risk of stroke among people who snore loud. Worsening matters, researchers say, loud snorers might suffer diseases of the carotid artery that pumps oxygenated blood to the neck, head and brain.

Some researchers believe that the vibrations caused by snoring disturb red blood cells as they pass through blood vessels through the throat. These disturbances, in turn, might cause negative impacts on blood vessels—inflaming arterial walls and damaging the body's ability to distribute or remove vital substances such as fats and cholesterol.

Despite all these various and potentially serious medical conditions, health professionals say that they consider normal snoring as a minor characteristic of the health process.

Nonetheless, at least judging by some accounts, relationships between spouses sometimes improve after one of them stops snoring—in some cases after doing so for extended periods of time, even following a number of years.

Discover vital methods to treat snoring

People worldwide, especially in America, go to great lengths to find medicines or devices designed to stop snoring.

A wide variety of devices sold via the Internet, through TV commercials and in print ads claim to guarantee they can stop this potentially bothersome affliction. Besides recommending weight loss and stop-smoking programs, many health experts stress the importance of using a variety of pillows or buying devices to insert into the mouth.

"The nurse sleeps sweetly, hired to watch the sick—whom snoring she disturbs," said William Cowper, an English poet who died in 1800 at age 68.

These days, many medical professionals urge consumers to seek the expert opinion or advice from a physician or a certified sleep-study center for expert advice.

Some sleep centers employ positive air pressure or CPAP machines to pump air into or out of the lungs. And certain devices strive to position the tongue or other areas of the mouth and neck in certain positions, in an effort to ensure a non-restricted air flow.

According to some published reports, only medical professionals can prescribe certain types of splints or devices designed to eliminate snoring. Some print advertisements or images promoting these appliances display images where splints keep the mouth open.

Consumers use a wide range of terms for such devices, from "jaw advancers" to "anti-snoring mouthpieces." Most of these devices strive to keep or maintain open space between the upper mouth and lower teeth to keep breathing airways unobstructed.

Ultimately, physicians stress the vital importance of getting a medical checkup, a prognosis and a possible recommendation before considering the use of such devices. Under continual medical care and prognosis, some patients even undergo surgery, as doctors strive to widen the throat's airways.
According to the "Stanford Online Report," some patients "slept

much more quietly" after physicians treated them using radio-frequency energy devices. The report said that doctors used the treatments to shrink the soft palate, thus widening the upper airway.

"The outpatient procedure, which proved safe with minimal side effects, shrank tissues in the mouth that can obstruct breathing during sleep," the report said.

The co-director of the Stanford Sleep Disorders Research Center, Dr. Nelson Powell, and his colleagues were quoted as saying that 22 people in the study experienced a 77 percent mean improvement on a standardized snoring scale and generally slept better.

Some media accounts describe the use of radio frequency ablation or RFA technology. Such systems use radiofrequency waves to remove tissue or tumors. For snorers, physicians sometimes use such devices to remove airway obstructions.

Meantime, vastly different possible solutions sometimes emerge for individuals who share a sleeping quarters with someone who snores. For them, potential solutions might range using earplugs to moving to a different bedroom.

An age-old proverb tells us that "when the river is deepest, it makes least noise." Perhaps unintentionally, American forefather Benjamin Franklin seemed to hit the mark dead-on target when he proclaimed "the worst wheel of the cart makes the most noise."

Certainly from the perspective of many people, excessive noise—particularly from snoring—can disturb the vital, urgent and necessary sleeping process. To many of these people, the need to find a solution to the snoring problem seems increasingly urgent.

CHAPTER 14

Enjoy a long, slow yawn

Have you ever heard stories about "traveling yawns?"

Under such scenarios, one person takes a long, deep yawn during a public event such as while listening to a church sermon amid a crowd of hundreds of people.

One or more individuals near this person see this initial yawn, and instinctively do the same. Before long, numerous other people within the same area start yawning as well.

Perhaps you've seen similar instances, everywhere from within classrooms to public transportation systems such as buses or subway cars. Many people swear such mimicked behavior invariably emerges, even when subsequent people fail to realize what's happening.

"Never yawn in front of a lady," said Frank Sinatra, a legendary American singer and actor who died in 1998 at age 82. Even the great "bard" William Shakespeare proclaimed some 400 years ago that "Tis now the very witching time of night, when churchyards yawn and hell itself breathes out contagion to this world."

Although many of us readily acknowledge such insights, though, just what is a yawn? Why do we naturally undergo such biological functions, and why do they seem to spread from person to person?

Medical experts insist that such reflexive action naturally occurs as the body's way to show tiredness, express boredom, and to stimulate the body or to stretch taught muscles. Invariably a yawn serves as a precursor to sleep, almost as if a necessary or close sibling of this vital resting process.

According to the Princeton University Press, expert research has confirmed that people often instinctively yawn when seeing someone else do that same. Some people have even gone so far as to claim that monkeys or chimps yawn after seeing creatures from the same species display such behavior.

Did you ever hide a yawn?

Have you ever been talking with someone face-to-face, when you felt overcome by an intense or deep need to take a long, deep yawn?

Faced with such a predicament, some people apparently fight back this instinctive and natural behavior—in a desperate attempt to avoid offending the other person.

"What if Hal thinks he's boring me to tears," Juanita might think, while fighting back a desperate need to yawn while talking to him. She covers her mouth, her eyes welling up with tears, cupping a hand to her mouth and pushing air through her ears.

The mere thought of such a predicament, or even the very sight of such a scene, might drive an observer to laughter. Even so, such a scenario might seem harrowing to anyone caught in such a scenario.

All along, some people claim that the body strives to yawn due to a lack of an adequate oxygen supply in the surrounding environment. However, an article in "American Scientist" reportedly has disputed the validity of such claims.

Specific possible reasons vary widely, as observers blame or cite a wide range of potential causes. While some people insist that yawns strive to relieve stress, others point to the body's need for cooling after exercise or to regulate the brain's glucose supplies.

From the perspective of many people, yawning seems closely related to the overall sleep process. We often yawn right before or shortly after long periods of rest. Still others insist that neurotransmitters within the brain generate yawning as responses to a wide variety of a person's physical needs—ranging from appetite to moods.

Theories on yawning seem inconclusive

Judging by the many diverse theories about the process of yawning, this biological process seems just as mysterious to medical experts as sleep itself.

Indeed, for thousands of years, some of the most knowledgeable teachers have proclaimed or described the so-called wonders of the world from the pyramids of Egypt to statue of Zeus at Olympia. Yet the mysteries of sleep and even of yawning have remained just as awe-inspiring.

To be sure, despite recent major advances in technology, from electronics-related developments such as the Internet to the Human Genome Project, the experts still lack a clear-cut cure for the common cold and they still lack a definitive answer for why we yawn.

Within such research, some of the greatest focus seems to have targeted the nagging question of why even the mere thought of yawning often makes us want to do that, let alone vivid images of the eyes or mouths of people undergoing such activity.

Various reports listed in a wide variety of publications or studies cite everything from the basic "herd instinct" prevalent in animal behavior to an innate or in-bred need to mimic those of the same species.

In fact, this basic need has become so intense that the urge to yawn can and does move among species, at least according to various news reports. The BBC News cited a study from Birkbeck College at the University of London, concluding that in laboratory studies dogs often yawned when people did the same in front of them.

"The team found that 21 out of 29 dogs yawned, when the (human) stranger in front of them yawned," the BBC said.

Meantime, such research apparently fails to ward off a nagging long-held belief, superstition or fear that our souls might escape or wander away when we yawn. According to the "Dictionary of Superstitions" published by Oxford University Press, some Christians have made the sign of the cross over their mouths when yawning.

Blinking also can signal sleep

Do you ever think about how often your eyes blink?

By some accounts, an average adult blinks about 9,600 times per day, or about 600 times per hour or 10 times per minute while awake.

Without us needing to think about the process, the body naturally and automatically dictates this activity to moisten the eyes, keeping them from becoming dirty or irritated.

Some researchers tell us that people generally blink less often while their eyes focus on a specific object for extended periods, such as while reading.

Conversely, medical professionals also say that an individual person blinks more when his or her eyes or body becomes fatigued. Thus, while the age-old saying tells us that "the eyes are mirrors of the soul," the amount of blinking might possibly indicate the degree or level that a person needs to sleep.

Herein rests another mystery, since infants usually blink much less often than adults, only about twice per minute compared to about 10 times per minute for maturing people. "The Register" online service reports that the rate of blinking increases as we age, possibly due to changes in sleep patterns.

Some published reports also indicate that additional stress as we age into our teens and beyond, coupled with changes in how we focus on the world, might play a significant role in these transitions.

Whatever the case, you might want to remain aware that when you see someone blink rapid-fire or with great frequency during short periods or when you do that as well, sleep might occur soon.

Super brain activity occurs during sleep

Within many cultures worldwide, physicians can legally declare a person dead when his or her brain waves stop functioning.

Brain waves occur when that organ transmits vital and necessary electrical impulses. Amazingly, at least from the perspective of many people, the brain and its electrical functions remain active even while we sleep. Absent brain waves denote death.

"When you fish for love, bait your heart—not your brain," said Mark Twain, the world-famous American author and humorist who died in 1910 at age 74.

Everyone from people with high IQs to folks with low intelligence depends on healthy brain function to continue while sleeping, vital in order to maintain good health. A person's overall vibrancy and mental acuity goes haywire when brain activity gets off kilter. In some cases seizures may be triggered by abnormal brain waves.

Otherwise negative symptoms like a chronic neurological disorder called epilepsy might occur, possibly resulting in potentially debilitating seizures. Other potential problems when brain waves go haywire range from migraine headaches to delirium or chronic periods of fainting.

Without dispute, the body fails to function and all its many trillions of cells would die without healthy brain wave activity, especially while we're asleep. Scientists say a wide variety of factors can cause or trigger abnormal or unhealthy brain wave patterns. these range from benign or malignant tumors to stokes or aneurisms.

Brain waves play a vital role in your sleep

Scientists tell us that brain wave activity during periods of rapid-eye-movement or REM sleep displays characteristics that appear somewhat similar to measurements of those patterns while we're awake. And remember, the REM stage of sleep remains vital to good health, largely because our bodies produce the greatest levels of human growth hormones while the eyes move rapidly during periods of deep rest.

Neurologists, physicians who specialize in nervous system disorders, measure brain waves by using EEG—or electroencephalography—machines that chart the brain's production of electrical activity. These measurements seek to identify vital health factors ranging from tumors to comas, seizures   and signs of a stroke.

From the standpoint of sleep, an EEG measures the brain's varying levels of electrical activity during all the various phases of rest—including REM sleep periods and amid so-called "slow-wave" sleep times while the eyes remain relatively calm.

These medical procedures often emerge as vital in related testing called PSG—or polysomnography—which physicians use to determine the quality of an individual's sleep. Medical professionals and certain sleep disorder facilities use PSG tests to diagnose a person's specific sleep problems and also to develop suggested treatments.

According to an article that first appeared in "Science" magazine in 1953, professors and graduate students at the University of Chicago first determined the significance of REM sleep during the early 1950s.

Besides monitoring brain activity during sleep, some sleep centers or physicians also simultaneously use other measuring devices to chart heart, eye and muscle activities. Some physicians and sleep experts apparently believe all these various bodily functions interact while we're asleep, partly in order to optimize good health.

In conducting these tests, called polysomnograms, physicians, medical professionals or staff members attach at least 20 or more wires to the patient's body. The systems monitor everything from the body's absorption of oxygen to how much the legs move during sleep. Some systems also record the sound levels of snoring, oxygen levels within the blood, and also vital bodily functions such as pulse rates.

CHAPTER 15

The profound, mysterious and seemingly magic process of dreaming

Since recorded history began, scientists, researchers, physicians and even people proclaiming to be psychics have admitted that they fail to fully understand the mysteries of dreams.

Even today, some doctors and sleep researchers confess that medical professionals still fail to assimilate all the varied and complex intricacies of the dreaming process. Nonetheless, researchers have concluded that our most intense and vivid dreams invariably occur during periods of rapid eye movement.

This holds significant meaning for medical professionals who insist dreams play an essential role in the healthy process that sleep makes possible. From a health standpoint, scientists refer to the study and research of dreams as oneirology.

According to the "Journal of Experimental Psychology," dreams experienced during the REM phase of sleep emerge as much more vivid and memorable than amid non-REM sleep. This seems significant from the perspective of some sleep researchers, largely because during the vast majority of sleep the eyes remain relatively calm.

In a 2007 article, "Brain Basics: Understanding Sleep" for the National Institute of Neurological Disorders and Stroke, researchers concluded that an average person undergoes about two hours of dreaming per night. According to some published reports, most dreams last only 5-20 minutes.

Logic tells at least some of us that an individual apparently must experience intense REM-period dreams, since that's the time frame when the body generates vital growth hormones.

Amid these so-called nightly shows within the brain, the bodies of healthy people perform amazing fetes, apparently in order to prevent the limbs from mimicking activities that would mirror our activities during "stories" or dreams that play out within the brain. During intense dreams, neurotransmitters course through the body, suppressing or shutting down the movement of certain muscles.

Dreams play a vital role in our memories

Perhaps most important, dreams apparently play a vital role in enabling the brain to generate or maintain vital long-term memories—functions necessary later during times when we're awake.

An age-old saying tells us to live so that memories will be part of our happiness. From a biological standpoint, such outcomes could only become possible thanks to sleep and dreams.

Jeremy Irons, an Academy Award®-winning film and stage actor born in England in 1948, has been quoted as saying that, "We all have our time machines. Some take us back, they're called memories. Some take us forward, they're called dreams."

Such eternal words of wisdom seem at least in some ways to mirror the conclusions of Sigmund Freud, the late famed psychiatrist. By numerous accounts, Freud's theories linked long-term memories and the dreaming process to the subconscious mind. This famed Austrian once humorously proclaimed: "The mind is like an iceberg. It floats with one-seventh of its bulk above water."

Within the limitations of what we know, some studies have concluded that many dreams get crammed with illogical occurrences. Numerous researchers insist this serves as the brain's ingenious method of solidifying the most deep and important memories, those involving integral cognitive functions ranging from interpretive meanings to understanding life's lessons.

In an October 2001 "Science" magazine article, researchers noted a reduction in the flow of information among various areas of the brain amid REM sleep. The scientists concluded that an increase in certain hormones during the rapid-eye-movement phase of rest generates a slowdown in the transmission of data within the mind.

"The brain is wider than the sky," wrote Emily Dickinson, an American poet who died in 1886 at age 55. Such observations seem on track to those of us who appreciate the importance of the dreaming process, particularly when considering and acknowledging the vital role that sleep plays throughout our entire lives.

Diverse theories abound involving dreams

Judging at least partly from the many diverse publications and articles about reasons for dreams, theories on what causes them seem as numerous as grains of sand on a beach.

"The human soul is hospitable and will entertain conflicting sentiments and contradictory opinions with much impartiality," said Mary Anne Evans, an English novelist who wrote under the penname George Eliot; she died in 1880 at age 61.

The seemingly endless stream of hypotheses or theories on why dreams occur range from an internal need to regulate moods to an apparent emotional desire to fulfill our fantasies. A 1964 article in "New Scientist" suggested that dreams might serve as the body's way of removing unnecessary information, similar in a sense to the way that computers eliminate certain data during the restart process.

Woody Allen, the legendary American film comic and writer born in 1935, seemed to find the proverbial needle in this haystack when quoted as saying, "In Beverly Hills, they don't throw their garbage away. They make it into television shows."

When accounting for such humor, we can also take solace in such observations as that by analytical psychologist Carl Jung, who noted in a 1948 article in "Princeton University Press"—13 years before dying in 1961 at age 85—of his belief that dreams enable an individual to compensate for his or her one-sided attitudes.

"Everything that irritates us about others can lead us to an understanding about ourselves," said Jung, who explored his in-depth theory or hypothesis that deep down human beings are "by nature religious."

Other observers or researchers have surmised that perhaps in a sense when describing our dreams to other people, we often end up discussing personal inner feelings or sensations that would otherwise go unspoken.

"Good communication is as stimulating as black coffee, and just as hard to sleep afterward," said Anne Morrow Lindbergh, the late author and aviator.

Others have even surmised that dreams enable us to create new concepts or ideas, perhaps as our minds sort out and discard useless information. Added to this comes a concept suggesting that perhaps dreams serve as an excellent mental coping mechanism, similar in some ways to psychoanalysis.

Dreams might relive potentially harmful stress

Ultimately, dreams might play an integral role in enabling our minds or nervous systems to lower or cope with potentially harmful stress, at least according to numerous research articles and clinical studies.

Still another age-old adage or common saying tells us that "stress is when you wake up screaming and realize you haven't fallen asleep yet." Some hypothesis even go so far as to suggest that dreams enable us to test or even re-test the validity or effectiveness of certain emotions, while in the same process abandoning certain possibilities as unhelpful.

Such analytical theories have even led various researchers to study how the mind discerns what is "realistic" between our dream world and so-called reality. Perhaps some of us fail to fully differentiate between dreams and our time awake, resulting in hallucinations or behaviors that many observers consider unhealthy.

By some accounts, Jung suggested that a person who acts out the same behaviors from his or her dreams might somehow suffer a deterioration of cognitive skills—possibly resulting in schizophrenia or other psychotic disorders.

Due partly to these reasons, some researchers believe that many people naturally crave sleep during extremely stressful life experiences as an internal and mental coping mechanism. Those who embrace such assumptions might argue that many psychotic people experience difficulty at fully benefiting from normal, healthy sleep.

Once again, such assumptions acknowledge the importance of sleep's vital and necessary role in eliminating or lessening potentially unhealthful stress.

"If you ask what is the single most important key to longevity, I would have to say it is avoiding worry, stress and tension," said George Burns, a legendary American comedian, writer and actor who died in 1996 at age 100. "And if you didn't ask me, I'd still have to say it."

Consider the meaning of dreams

Seemingly since time began, people and various cultures have developed a wide range of theories about what specific dreams mean.

While some observers might insist a certain dream evolved as a direct result of divine or heavenly intervention, another person might insist the same experience emerged from a biological or chemical-related process.

Various spiritual beliefs or religions consider specific dreams as divine, inspirational messages from God. Some believers even strive to make their dreams evolve or transform into only good or positive experiences.

Under such intense scrutiny, perhaps dreams serve as merely each person's way of expressing his or her most intense cravings or worries, as Jung once suggested.

The difficulty or challenge of discerning between the dream world and reality became a persistent theme in the late Rod Serling's anthology series "The Twilight Zone," with initial episodes airing on American TV from 1959-1964.

Amid our deepest, healthiest and most profound sleep, certainly many dreams delve into our most profound emotions and desires. Throughout many cultures such deeply personal subjects might involve subjects considered socially taboo or even forbidden and unlawful, such as intensive or highly orgasmic sex.

"Our life is composed greatly from dreams, from the unconscious, and they must be brought into connection with action. They must be woven together," said Anaïs Nin, a French-born American writer of journals, famous for her erotica; she died 1977 at age 73.

Amid such observations, dreams—and the sleeping process that makes them possible—force us to acknowledge that as human beings and mammals we're animals, each packed with natural and powerful biological cravings and emotional desires.

Partly as a result, many researchers express little surprise in various studies that indicate people from extremely different cultures and religions worldwide often experience similar content or stories in their dreams. Such frequent, persistent and common bonds give hope among many of the world's greatest thinkers and to those who have taught us about the urgent and vital need for sharing.

"An individual cannot start living until he can rise above the narrow confines of his individualistic concerns to the broader concerns of all humanity," said the Rev. Dr. Martin Luther King Jr., an American clergyman and civil rights activist killed by an assassin in 1968 at age 39.

Dreams provide an emotional release

Researchers tell us that dreams provide an essential means for releasing or venting intense emotions. For this reason, psychiatrists express little surprise when people proclaim that negative feelings or sensations dominate their dreams, far surpassing instances where positive emotions might seem prevalent.

"A man who is a master of himself can end a sorrow as easily as he can invent a pleasure," said Oscar Wilde, an Irish playwright and author who died in 1900 at age 46. "I don't want to be at the mercy of my emotions. I want to use them, to enjoy them, and to dominate them."

Indeed, at least judging from what some researchers have concluded, dreams might at least in part or perhaps in a very large sense enable us to control or manage our most intense emotions—ranging from anger to feelings of extreme love, loss or grief.

With little wonder, then, sleep experts also chronicle clinical results which indicate that many people experience recurring dreams. Possibly in order to deal with certain stresses or to re-experience pleasurable events, a majority of people often dream of the same stories or similar events.

Topics might cover a vastly diverse range, everything from getting caught naked in a public place to using the arms as if wings in order to fly. These topics often delve deep into our individual desires or cravings, on a spiritual or physical level.

Tori Amos, a British-born American singer and songwriter born on 1963, has been quoted as saying that "I think you have to know who you are. Get to know the monster that lives within your soul, dive deep into your soul, and explore it."

Embracing such philosophies, from ancient Greek societies through the present day, many people have specialized in trying to interpret dreams. This process entails deciphering specifics of each dream, while reaching conclusions on what message each such experience might convey.

Some dreams emerge "below the rainbow"

In the classic 1939 movie "The Wizard of Oz," the main character Dorothy lives in a state depicted as black-and-white — Kansas.

After a flying window frame blown by a horrific tornado knocks Dorothy unconscious, she dreams of landing above a rainbow in a wonderful, color-filled land called Oz. Many dreams give a similar sense of magic at least in scenes involving color.

According to researchers, some people experience dreams in black-and-white. The percentages of dreamers who fail to experience the sensation of color seem to vary, depending on the study involved.

Complicating matters, at varying stages in life most people suffer from nightmares, those extremely unpleasant or horrific dreams. Some nightmares occur as a result of traumatic life experiences or due to physical reactions from health problems, sleep researchers say.

"When one creates phantoms for oneself, one puts vampires into the world, and one must nourish these children of a voluntary nightmare with one's blood—one's life—one's intelligence and one's reason, without ever satisfying them," said Eliphas Lévi, a French magician and occult author who died in 1875 at age 65.

Needless to say, even amid nourishing and life-giving sleep, hellish dreams can make the world seem threatening and untenable. Some mind-bending nightmares involve torture or suspenseful struggles to escape almost certain death or horrific injury.

Eager to conquer bouts of persistent and nagging nightmares, some researchers suggest trying to develop "lucid dreams"—where the dreamer remains fully cognizant that he or she is undergoing a dream, while striving to control the actions involved within the story.

Experience orgasms during dreams

Medical professionals tell us that a fulfilling sex life among consenting adults serves a vital and necessary role in helping people achieve and maintain good health—just as powerful of an urge or desire as sleep.

Thus, sleep researchers find little surprise in discovering what many people and cultures have already known instinctively and through natural experience for thousands of years. On occasion, healthy adults experience orgasms or "wet dreams" while sleeping.

The percentage of our dreams featuring sexual content seems to vary, depending on the research involved. While many healthy adults never experience such sensations during sleep, some individuals undergo—or even enjoy—spontaneous dreams that involve intense sexual experiences.

According to researchers, "nocturnal emissions" while dreaming seem more prevalent among teens and young adults, a period in life when certain sex-related and growth hormones surge.

"Sensuality often makes love grow too quickly, so that the root remains weak and is easy to pull out," said Friedrich Nietzsche, a widely acclaimed German philosopher who died in 1900 at age 55.

Even for dreams that lack sexual connotations, for thousands of years in many diverse cultures people have looked to their sleep-period dreams as potential sources for inspiration. Whether dreams instill within us a need or demand for personal responsibility apparently remains a matter for philosophers to continue pondering, perhaps for many generations to come.

Ultimately, the overall function of dreams might generate a peaceful state of mind, perhaps sensations of contentment or tranquility. Many of us consider sleep as a non-ruffled, care-free state, at least when experienced in ideal or preferred conditions.

"Happiness is the meaning and the purpose of life, the whole aim and end of human existence," said Aristotle, the Greek philosopher who lived more than 300 years before Christ. For those of us who embrace and appreciate the many benefits of sleep, such observations acknowledge the need for a comfortable setting within humanity's continual quest for happiness.

Those many "forgettable" dreams

Despite the vital significance of dreams to the sleeping process, many of us invariably forget the details of a vast majority of those experiences—seemingly from the very moment we awaken. Unless we make conscious attempts to recall specifics of our dreams, such details often flutter from memory as if new-fallen leaves in a stiff autumn breeze.

By some accounts, men fail to recall specific details of dreams more frequently than women, who generally possess a greater recollection of this information. Adding even more to the mystery, some dreams involve so-called "real life" sensations as they occur, such as hearing an ambulance siren within a dream—at the same moment that such a vehicle passes on a nearby street while we sleep.

Amid this interaction between the boundaries of our conscious and unconscious realms, we sometimes use dream states as transitions for the mind, researchers say.

Beginning from early childhood many of us learned of an age-old prayer that some of our parents encouraged or demanded that we say at bedtime. While specific wording might vary among versions, the basic message remains:

> Now I lay me down to sleep
> I pray the Lord my soul to keep
> N' if I die before I awake
> I pray the Lord my soul to take

Without question, whatever an individual's particular belief system, the sleeping and dreaming process somehow seem to place us closer to the creator—or at least our individual versions of some sort of unseen protector.

For such morals or perceptions to hold any significant value, we must always seize the opportunity to sleep in as restful and placid a manner as possible. Our chances for continued good health in both a spiritual and a physical sense could very well depend on such an attitude throughout your lifetime.

CHAPTER 16

Sleep involves vital stages throughout life

Starting while in our mothers' wombs, and lasting till the day we die—hopefully in old age—the sleep process evolves and changes throughout life.

Infants up to one month old typically sleep 18 hours daily, while babies from a month old to 12 months snooze 14-18 hours each day, according to sleep experts. The need for shut-eye gradually tapers off, from 12-15 hours daily from ages 1-3, and then down to 9-10 hours during the teenage years.

Physicians recommend that adults including seniors get 7-8 hours sleep each day, while pregnant women often should sleep at least nine hours or more.

"Many things—such as loving, going to sleep, or behaving unaffectedly—are done worst when we try hardest to do them," said Edgar Watson Howe, an American editor and novelist who died in 1937 at age 84.

While benefiting our overall health, sleep also improves the memory and makes people more alert, decreasing the probability of mishaps, according to the National Sleep Foundation.

At all stages of life, each sleep session involving a multi-hour period has three primary stages. The first phase involves drowsiness and brain wave patterns ranging from alpha to theta, or spanning the range from 4-13 on the hertz or "Hz" scale. Around half our sleep time involves the next deeper scale, in the 12-16 Hz range when the individual loses any sense of his or her surroundings.

Finally, within the deepest sleep scale of 0.5-4 Hz, sometimes referred to as "slow-wave sleep," the brain experiences what scientists call delta waves—which occurs about half the time while we sleep.

A wide range of mysterious or difficult-to-understand sleep disorders can occur during deep sleep. Such abnormalities or levels of parasomnia can involve a wide spectrum of bodily functions, impacting everything from emotions to limb movements. Some of the most specific or prevalent potential problems include:

● **Sleep-talking**: People speak aloud during sleep, sometimes even lengthy, drawn-out speeches. Some sleep-talking episodes occur on numerous occasions during a single sleep session, potentially bothering other individuals. According to some published reports, people listening to sleep-talkers might have difficulty deciphering what the sleeper says. By some accounts, half of children talk during sleep at least on occasion, a characteristic many children outgrow in their teens.

● **Bedwetting**: Past the age when most toddlers or children learn to control their bladders while asleep, some children and older adults urinate while they snooze. Many sleep experts insist that parents often worry too much, making a bigger deal than necessary, about the bedwetting of any child over ages 7-8. While the propensity of such symptoms might stem at least partly from heredity, a vast majority of people ages 10 and older manage to refrain from bedwetting. Those who wet the bed sometimes experience negative psychological impacts, partly hinged on how other people respond to the situation.

● **Night terrors**: These sleepers suffer extreme terror while asleep, often experiencing difficulty in attempts to awaken. Some people with this condition begin screaming or make other gut-wrenching sounds when suddenly awakened from deep sleep, especially aroused during the rapid-eye-movement phase. Unlike nightmares, during night terrors the person suffers adverse symptoms while not fully asleep. Some researchers believe an individual's specific emotions trigger these horrific episodes.

● **Sleepwalking**: People suffering from this condition, while fully asleep, sometimes walk around performing everyday activities, at least judging by some eyewitness accounts. Sleep experts say many of the people who exhibit such behavior have high levels of stress. In 1997, the Neurology.org Web site reported that children comprise the vast majority of sleepwalkers. Some seemingly unbelievable reports insist that numerous sleepwalkers have driven cars, danced or even committed murder while asleep. According to some researchers, an unknown number of "sleepwalkers" unknowingly engage in sexual intercourse while sleeping.

● **Sleep-related eating disorder**: Sometimes called "night eating disorder" or NED, this condition usually involves what medical professionals call "late-night binge eating." These people sometimes awaken—or while still groggy from sleep—only to gorge themselves with extreme amounts of food.

● **Sleep paralysis**: The body either becomes or seems paralyzed, particularly during REM or rapid-eye-movement sleep. Some researchers believe that during REM sleep, in healthy people the body essentially undergoes a period of paralysis. However, when people suffering symptoms of sleep paralysis awaken during REM sleep, some portions or all of their bodies continue exhibiting the characteristics of paralysis. Even after awakening, such symptoms might last for several minutes—potentially causing the person to panic.

● Narcolepsy: People suffering from this condition sometimes go to sleep suddenly during the daytime with little or no warning. Often overwhelmed by severe drowsiness during the day, these individuals often experience serious health hazards. People with narcolepsy sometimes unknowingly endanger others by falling asleep while driving or amid other inappropriate activities. Amazingly, this condition can occur while talking, and—yes—even during sexual activity.

● **Insomnia**: Suffering from perhaps one of the most common sleep disorders, people with this condition experience difficulty falling asleep or staying asleep. According to an article published by the National Institute of Neurological Disorders and Stroke, at least 64 million Americans suffer from insomnia on a regular basis at least once each year. This situation becomes worse for women, whom some researchers believe experience insomnia nearly 1 _ times more often than men. Researchers cite dozens of potential causes, ranging from drugs, caffeine and parasites to brain lesions, neurological disorders and abusing non-prescription sleep drugs. In addition, menopausal insomnia may occur with lowered levels of progesterone hormones. In fact, according to some studies, losing just one hour of sleep each night can increase the risk of heart attacks by up to 30 percent.

● **Fatal familial insomnia**: Those with this very rare hereditary fatal brain disease progressively find sleeping impossible until they eventually die. Symptoms usually begin from ages 30-60, but most often after 50 years old. As a result, people with this condition unknowingly can pass this characteristic on to their offspring, with each newborn reportedly having a 50 percent chance of getting the disease—instilled within their bodies before birth.

● **Restless legs syndrome**: Most people with this condition—often called "RLS"—get a seemingly uncontrollable urge to move various parts of their bodies such as the arms or legs. Some sufferers tell physicians they get temporary relief from some of the worst symptoms by moving the affected body parts, after experiencing uncomfortable sensations such as itching in those areas of the body. These problems, in turn, often cause difficulty sleeping. Dozens of potential or suspected causes range from iron deficiencies to hereditary factors. This symptom may accompany obstructive sleep apnea.

- **Delayed sleep-phase syndrome**: The timing of the internal biological clock goes haywire in people with this condition, adversely affecting sleep patterns and their abilities to become or remain alert during peak periods of the day. Many people with this syndrome consider awakening difficult in the morning, often after remaining awake well past midnight.

- **Advanced sleep phase syndrome**: Despite their efforts to change personal sleep patterns, people with this condition fall asleep very early in the evening, and awaken many hours before sunrise.

- **Bruxism**: Commonly called "teeth grinding," this condition's most notable characteristics involve the clinching of the jaw while asleep—often damaging the teeth or dental area if the condition persists over extended periods.

- **Nocturia**: This condition forces a person to awaken one or several times each night in order to urinate. Individual cases of nocturia might indicate the incidence of other medical problems including prostate cancer, chronic renal failure, benign prostate, hypertrophy, diabetes, urinary bladder disease or several other conditions.

- **Nocturnal myoclonus**: Even amid deep REM-level sleep, people suffering from this condition involuntarily move their arms and legs in various directions. Needless to say, besides disturbing these individuals, their bed partners often get bothered—potentially disrupting their own sleep as well, or even injuring their bed partners.

● **Non-24 hour sleep-wake syndrome**: Among the rarest sleep disorders, this forces an individual to go to sleep up to a few hours earlier than had been done the day before. This pattern continues daily for a few weeks, until eventually the individual completes the cycle—which then continues without letup.

● **Obesity hypoventilation syndrome**: Often called "Pickwickian syndrome," this condition most often afflicts seriously overweight people. When sleeping, their breathing problems cause carbon dioxide levels to get too high in the blood, which fails to receive adequate oxygen supplies.

● **Ondine's curse**: Considered fatal if left untreated, this condition involves a respiratory disorder during sleep—when breathing could stop. Out of every one million children who are born, an estimated five of them suffer from this condition, also called congenital central hypoventilation syndrome. Sometimes trauma to the brainstem generates this condition.

● **Sleeping sickness**: Sometimes called or affiliated with "lethargy" or "fatigue," this condition has been referred to by a wide variety of names or terms. Occasionally labeled as "exhaustion," in general laymen's terms this condition afflicts a person who has continued moving or working past his or her ability to perform. Rather than listing fatigue as an illness, some physicians or sleep experts label such occurrences as symptoms of other physical or mental conditions.

● **Other disorders**: The many other disorders include sleep apnea—the condition where people intermittently stop breathing while asleep—and excessive, loud or potentially bothersome snoring.

Physicians and scientists list a wide variety of other sleep disorders and also of apparent causes, plus just as many potential remedies or possible solutions for these many afflictions. If left untreated, such conditions could result in adverse health or ultimately even death.

Each specific type of sleep disorder involves a certain type of suggested remedy or medication that only an allopathic physician, homeopath, acupuncturist, psychiatrist or other medical professional can recommend.

Heed advice from health experts

All serious sleep disorders require treatment from certified, licensed medical professionals. Only these people possess qualifications necessary to diagnose and treat apparent problems that involve your need to snooze.

While the need to sleep and the process of engaging in such activity often comes naturally to most people, the lay person should avoid relying on "wives' tales and quack remedies." Any attempt to diagnose or treat ourselves might exacerbate the condition, or even result in additional health problems.

Voltaire, a French writer and philosopher during the Enlightenment who died in 1778 at age 83, missed the mark when he quipped—perhaps humorously: "Doctors are men who prescribe medicines of which they know little, to cure diseases of which they know less, in human beings of which they know nothing."

To the contrary, unlike perhaps hundreds of years ago, today's physicians have made tremendous strides during the past 50 years, particularly in matters involving sleep. Although much still remains unknown about the snoozing process, tremendous strides in research have enabled doctors to develop solutions, many of them unheard of in the mid-1950s.

The beloved movie comic actor Walter Matthau, who died in 2000 at age 79, joked that, "My doctor once gave me six months to live, but when I couldn't pay the bill he gave me six months more." Embracing such philosophies, many people adhere to a longtime saying telling us that "just because your doctor has a name for your condition, doesn't mean he knows what it is."

Slapping such negative convictions in the face, anyone suspected of suffering from a serious sleep disorder or who is related to that individual, should face such matters with serious resolve. These people should follow such strategies, however comical a specific condition might seem, such as sleepwalking or sleep-talking. After all, knowing the basics might very well save your life.

Life's everyday hassles hamper sleep

Every day seemingly countless people worldwide find themselves struck with sudden tragedies that prevent them from getting adequate sleep.

Besides wars, horrific storms, earthquakes and other natural disasters, unexpected nasty emails or news of a sudden death in the family can prevent adequate rest. These situations, in turn, might lead to a sudden decline in overall good health.

Researchers say the very nature of sleep enables us to at least partly resolve or cope with potential or ongoing stressful situations. Any event that threatens or eliminates sleep hinders the body's natural processes.

As a so-called first line of defense, some health experts recommend that everyone adopt steady and reliable "sleep hygiene" habits. Medical professionals who embrace such strategies believe that people who become overly sleepy during the day or who experience difficulty sleeping sometimes fail to follow established sleep patterns and routines.

At least one celebrity or widely known personality has been quoted as saying that "the secret of your future is hidden in your daily routine." In sharp contrast to those who proclaim that boring routine can lead to an early death, still others insist that healthy and regular regimens such as good exercise and sleep habits can energize our lives.

Along these lines, those who embrace or recommend good sleep hygiene tell us to eat in moderation before sleep and to carefully time or plan for sleep. The process involves everything from going to bed at a consistent, predictable time each day to working beforehand to assure a comfortable or relaxing environment. This way, they insist we can generate or establish productive and predictable lifestyle patterns.

Sleep occurs on a massive scale

Assuming that an average individual sleeps about eight hours daily, at any given moment, one third of the more than 6 billion people on earth are fast asleep.

That means as you read this page, a whopping 2 billion people are now sleeping in a wide variety of conditions from extremely hot environments to very cold conditions. Like you probably do, a vast majority of them strive to get as comfortable as possible for snooze time.

Confucius, the great Chinese thinker and philosopher more than 400 years before Christ, claimed that, "The superior man thinks always of virtue; the common man thinks of comfort."

But many of today's medical professionals might beg to differ, especially considering what researchers now know about the many benefits of remaining comfortable in order to achieve and maintain healthful rest.

Without question all of today's more than 6 billion human inhabitants on Earth eventually will die, hopefully the vast majority of them from natural causes. And while overall research might remain inclusive, odds seem strong that people who get the most comfortable, least-stressful rest will enjoy longer, more fulfilling lives.

"A man 90 years old was asked to what he attributed his longevity," observed Garson Kanin, an American writer and director who died in 1999 at age 86. "I reckon he said, with a twinkle in his eye, 'It was because most nights I went to bed and slept when I should have sat up and worried.'"

For now, the many mysterious and diverse causes of a wide variety of pervasive sleep disorders might range from chemical imbalances within individuals to bothersome or difficult-to-detect forces such as food allergies.

While the world's top physicians and sleep centers work to pinpoint specific problems and to develop solutions, collectively and individually we should strive to do our best in assuring the most restful and restorative sleep for ourselves.

CHAPTER 17

Lack of sleep generates immune prolems

"Don't you dare go outside without a coat on, or you'll catch a cold," many mothers have warned their children, worried about such potential results.

Interestingly, however, although our parents might have urged or demanded that we get plenty of sleep as children, only a small percentage of adults seem to realize the important role that sleep plays in strengthening and in maintaining our immune systems.

While sleep provides a vital, necessary and important role in healing injuries, all along a lack of adequate snooze time could weaken our bodies' abilities to ward off or fight illness, according to some research.

A 2007 report in "Pediatrics" described a study where rats suffered weakened immune systems after researchers deprived the animals of sleep for 24-hour periods. As compared to a control group allowed to sleep regular schedules, the levels of vital white blood cells that fight infections decreased 20 percent in sleep-deprived rats.

Animals deprived of sleep for more than seven days experience everything from open sores to loss of body mass and eventually death, according to a 223-page book first printed in 2003 by the same name of an organization that wrote it, "The Committee on Guidelines for the Use of Animals in Neuroscience and Behavioral Research."

Adding to the luster of sleep's solid overall reputation, a 2000 article in the "Journal of the American Medical Association" cited laboratory results that indicate men who experience greater percentages of slow-wave sleep also experience higher levels of growth hormone secretion into their bodies. Growth hormone is the "master hormone," the most important factor in the aging process.

"When we sleep well, we wake up feeling refreshed, alert and ready to face daily challenges," says National Sleep Foundation literature. "When we don't, every part of our lives can suffer. Our jobs, relationships, productivity, health and safety—and that of those around us—are all put at risk. And lack of sleep due to sleep loss and sleep disorders is taking a serious toll."

Nature generates two reasons for sleep

On a daily basis we see clocks tracking the minutes and seconds, displayed on everything from cell phones to computers and TV-timing devices.

Amazingly, though, few people seem to realize that our brains also possess and regulate internal biological clocks that help regulate when and how we decide to fall asleep. Physicians refer to this as the "circadian biological clock," an internal mechanism that automatically helps determine and regulate when our bodies become sleepy.

Thanks to this internal regulation system, certain organs and bodily functions fluctuate as necessary such as variations in kidney function or even blood pressure decreases.

Also, almost as if a rubber band that gets pulled to the breaking point on a child's wind-up toy airplane, we become sleepier the longer we remain awake. For us, the release of this built-up process comes when we allow ourselves to fall asleep.

Especially in more mature people, joint pain or discomfort caused by deteriorating muscles might tend to disrupt this natural process—perhaps making sleep difficult or seemingly impossible.

Jennifer Aniston, an American movie and TV star born in 1969, has been quoted as saying that "the greater your capacity to love, the greater your capacity to feel the pain." Those of us who embrace such philosophy should focus on the best, most natural and non-intrusive potential solutions when seeking effective methods for solving our sleep-related problems.

Listen to advice from experts

Embracing the importance of preparing and setting the mood for a good healthy snooze, the National Sleep Foundation gives numerous suggestions. Among them:

- **Caffeine**: During the final hours before scheduled sleep time, avoid foods or beverages that contain caffeine such as coffee, chocolate and soft drinks.

- **Nicotine**: Refrain from smoking cigarettes or chewing tobacco.

- **Exercise**: Maintain healthy and consistent exercise habits, but avoid strenuous activities within three hours before scheduled sleep time.

- **Routine**: Establish and maintain relaxing, stress-free activities regularly before bedtime such as soaking in a hot tub or taking a bath.

● **Environment**: Create or maintain an environment ideal for sleep, a dark and quiet place where you feel comfortable at a relaxing temperature.

Physicians and sleep experts emphasize the need to embrace and maintain such good-sleep tips, especially if you're among the estimated 20 million Americans who work at times other than during a standard 8 a.m. to 5 p.m. shift.

Know when to see a doctor

Remember that sleep researchers report that they have identified and continue to study what many people might consider a whopping 80 separate sleep disorders.

Even individuals who lack any of these potentially debilitating afflictions can suffer from sleep problems. Partly as a result, the National Sleep Foundation recommends that people who have difficulty sleeping maintain a "sleep diary," in order to chronicle specific details of their problems. Among potential conditions for observation:

● **Snoring**: Do people tell you that you shore loudly, or do you sometimes realize you're doing that?

● **Breathing**: Have people told you that you stop breathing for awhile during sleep, or have you even noticed this yourself?

● **Sudden sleep**: Have you suddenly or unexpectedly fallen asleep while undergoing regular daily activities such as driving a car, watching TV or reading?

● **Unpleasant sensations**: Do you experience creepy or strange sensations in your legs while sleeping or while attempting to fall asleep?

● **Sleep deprivation**: Are you frequently awakened by everything from pain or discomfort to noise, heartburn, bad dreams or a need to urinate.

For you, only a physician or medical professional can diagnose whether having any of these occurrences might cause reason for concern.

Consider natural solutions

Many people prefer to use or develop natural, non-drug solutions for their sleep-related problems. Potential remedies outside the pharmaceutical realm range from relaxation techniques to yoga or even moving into separate bedrooms—away from loud snorers.

A primary motive for seeking non-drug solutions stems from the fact that many people become dependant or addicted to pharmaceutical products designed to induce sleep.

Anyone suffering from sleep problems—but who wants to avoid drugs—should tell his or her doctor what natural, non-medicine treatments are already being used. And a doctor might suggest some or all these lifestyle choices after reaching a diagnosis. Among possible solutions that avoid standard medications:

● **Yoga**: This practice uses any one—or a combination of—mental and physical practices designed partly to put the body and mind in a relaxing state. There are numerous different types of yoga, and the goal of many practitioners entails spiritual matters—far more than merely striving to relax.

● **Biofeedback**: Considered a non-traditional or alternative form of medicine, this process involves developing a conscious awareness that practitioners say can control many bodily functions ranging from muscle tensions to heart rates and blood pressure. Many biofeedback systems utilize technology, enabling people to monitor their own physiological information.

● **Physical exercise**: While the overall goal usually involves achieving and maintaining a fit or healthy body, some people realize that briskly moving our muscles can produce tiredness—potentially resulting in sound sleep. However, remember that some researchers recommend avoiding exercise within three hours before scheduled sleep time.

● **Acupuncture**: Practitioners of this technique insert needles in various areas of the body for therapeutic purposes—including in some instances to aid in the sleep process, or in response to problems with sleeping.

● **Reflexology**: Sometimes called "zone therapy" for the improvement of general health, this involves manipulating the feet and sometimes the ears or hands.

● **Hypnosis**: On a serious level rather than as often depicted in TV or movie dramas and stage shows, this involves what some practitioners call a "wakeful state of focused attention." The hypnotherapy process involves people attempting to use hypnosis for therapeutic purposes, in efforts to modify behavior.

Once again, make sure a physician gives you a thorough checkup and authorizes the use of such measures. Medical professionals can suggest activities likely to generate the best results.

A scientist in his laboratory is not a mere technician," said Marie Curie, a Polish-born French physicist who died in 1934 at age 66. "He is also a child confronting natural phenomena that impress him as though they were fairy tales."

Certainly, since sleep by its very nature emerges as a complex process in the eyes of medical professionals, finding and honing the various potential solutions for related problems can become a hit-and-miss proposition.

Just as there is no known consistent cure for the common cold, we can safely proclaim that potential solutions for sleep disorders or problems remain diverse. For the most part, the perfect or ideal "recipe" for each individual's solutions might involve extensive testing or fine-tuning before ideal solutions can emerge.

"Every great and deep difficulty bears in itself its own solution," said Niels Bohr, a Danish physicist who died in 1962 at age 77. "It forces us to change our thinking in order to find it."

Establish specific and predictable routines

Before making a final decision on whether to pursue drugs as an option, people with sleep problems might want to consider regulating or manipulating their daily routines. These modifications could enable the body to establish and eventually maintain predictable sleep patterns. Among some of the most frequent options:

- **Slow down**: About one hour or so before your regular nightly bedtime, start slowing down your activities and go at a slower pace.

- **Routine**: Almost as if on a military regimen during military boot camp, awaken at the same time each day and go to bed at a pre-set hour each night.

- **Avoid stress**: Strive to refrain from thinking about employment responsibilities unless you're at the workplace. And if you work out of your home, avoid going into your personal workspace unless absolutely necessary.

- **Venting**: Talk to other people about things that cause you stress or briefly write down some of those feelings, in order to vent your emotions—rather than during the middle of the night when your body needs to sleep.

- **Environment**: Establish and maintain a quiet, safe and comfortable environment for sleep.

Ultimately, you should know best when and how to establish and maintain these various physical and environmental factors.

"Your mind will answer most questions if you learn to relax and wait for the answer," said William S. Burroughs, an American novelist, essayist, painter and social critic who died in 1997 at age 83.

CHAPTER 18

Consider the risks and rewards
Of sleep medications

Thanks to extensive research and development following many years of testing by lab technicians and physicians, medical professionals have developed many dozens of pharmaceutical products designed to bring us sleep.

Ranging from sedatives to common sleeping tablets, individually or in mixtures these drugs might bring desired results or create difficult-to-overcome additions—or even generate varying degrees of both outcomes.

From the start, keep in mind that certain drugs can generate a psychological dependence that becomes so powerful a person feels he or she can only sleep after using the medication. Thus, anyone considering the use of drugs should do so at the start with extreme caution, only after carefully considering the potential rewards and possible risks.

"Drugs are a bet with your mind," said Jim Morrison, an American singer, songwriter, poet and filmmaker who died in 1971 at age 27; some people contend he died from a heroin overdose, while others cite apparent heart problems.

Of course, as with all medications, people seeing to use medications to treat sleep problems should do so under the supervision and a prescription from a physician or other certified and licenses medical professional.

Many individuals might consider the potential use of drugs only as a last resort, partly because of the pervasive risk of adverse side affects. Also, people who get such prescriptions should take these medications only in the suggested manner.

Complicating matters, besides posing the risk of generating psychological dependence, some medications might generate an even more troublesome physical or biological need to retake the drug. All these various options pile up to create a proverbial roulette wheel, where users essentially take a gamble that a medication will generate desired results.

Realize potential dangers from the start

Many of the most seasoned physicians and medical professionals stress the urgent need to understand the grave dangers that certain sleep drugs might pose.

People using any of a wide variety of sleep medications run the risk of becoming involved in car crashes or even becoming too sleepy at inopportune times. As if to issue a vital warning sign, some research has indicated that certain sleep medications cause serious lifetime dependencies.

A new safer sedative called Rozerem® releases natural melatonin to aid sleep.

In addition, various specific sleep drugs including certain barbiturates are officially listed as narcotics, meaning that to possess, manufacture or distribute them without a prescription constitutes a felony—punishable by jail time and significant monetary fines.

"Caution is the eldest child of wisdom," said Victor Hugo, a French playwright and novelist who died in 1885 at age 83.

While well aware of these various severe potential dangers, some physicians choose to prescribe such medications anyway, largely in good-faith and while motivated by well-intended efforts to help their patients get much-needed sleep.

"The person who risks nothing, has nothing, does nothing, is nothing, and becomes nothing," said Leo Buscaglia, an author and motivational speaker who died in 1998 at age 74. "He may avoid suffering and sorrow, but he certainly cannot learn and feel and change and grow and love and live."

To this end, then, the ultimate decision on whether to use drugs for sleep problems involves a vital risk-verses-potential-reward situation—in which, ultimately, only the patient can make the vital decision on whether to start using such medications.

Learn about basic drug classifications

After diagnosing a specific sleep disorder, a licensed physician can consider issuing a prescription from a wide array of potential medications. Effective sedative agents should reduce anxiety, while exerting a calming effect with little or no impact on mental function or the body's motor skills.

From the perspective of most laymen, such pharmaceuticals are simply "drugs." But anyone serious about his or her sleep problem needs to know the primary basic types of narcotics, in order to understand potential risks and rewards. Herein you can review basic details of the primary types of sleep drug or options:

Benzodiazepine

Sometimes used for anti-anxiety purposes or as sedatives, this general class of drugs serves a psychoactive role—meaning that the medication primarily targets the central nervous system. This category contains the popular drugs Valium®, Ativan® and Serax® .

In the process, drugs within this class sometimes serve a "hypnotic" role, producing sleep. However, from the viewpoint of people seeking to treat sleep problems, drugs within this class also pose potentially unnecessary risks like dependence or addiction.

Physicians urge extreme caution, especially in instances were benzodiazepine medications might adversely impact a variety of other specific medical conditions ranging from pregnancy to psychosis.

Adding to the potential danger, even when prescribed in efforts to induce sleep, medications within this classification could induce adverse side affects including depression, amnesia, jaundice, weakness, trembling, headaches and confusion.

Worsening matters, some users—even those who have used such drugs for extended periods—sometimes suffer from severe withdrawal problems. The adverse and addictive nature of these drugs have motivated many nations worldwide to classify such medications as illegal unless possessed and distributed for purposes prescribed by physicians.

According to the National Law Enforcement Drug Research Fund, the many long-term adverse symptoms from extended use of benzodiazepines include dizziness, personality changes, dependence, aggression, irritability and nausea.

Non-benzodiazepines

Some researchers report or indicate that numerous drugs within this classification lack many of the potentially adverse side affects as benzodiazepines. All along, many of the pharmaceuticals within this class are sometimes deemed effective at inducing sleep.

However, just like benzodiazepines, medications within this class also carry the risk of potentially causing psychological dependence and physical dependence—potentially causing difficulties in attempts to stop using these drugs.

While dissimilar to benzodiazepines on a structural basis, these newer medications also pose the danger of creating addiction, especially when used for extended periods.

Just as distressing, non-benzodiazepines pose the risk of damaging or lessening a person's memory or cognitive abilities.

The many individual prescription medications within the imidazopyridines class of this category include Ambien®, Ambien CR®, Zolnod® and numerous others.

The other two primary classes are pyrazolopyrimidines, which include the trade name Sonata®, and cyclopyrrolones, that include the trade names Lunesta® and Imovane®. Sleep amnesia can emerge as a serious side effect of this drug class; some people suffering from sleep amnesia report they have gotten out of bed and driven cars at night while asleep—unaware of their dangerous activities until the following morning. Barbiturates such as Seconal®, Nembutal® and Phenobarbitol® are rarely used in modern medicine for sedation purposes.

Antidepressants

Besides drugs in the benzodiazepine and non-benzodiazepine classes, some physicians choose to prescribe antidepressant drugs in efforts to manage their patients' sleep or as an insomnia treatment.

Psychiatrists often employ antidepressant pharmaceuticals as an anti-psychotic medication, trying to alleviate the adverse impacts of significant depression.

The brand drugs in this classification range from Desyrl® to Risperdal® and many more. Pharmaceutical companies develop and test antidepressants designed as tranquilizers or sedatives, sometimes used to induce sleep-like conditions.

Off-label prescriptions

Physicians sometimes prescribe specific medications for off-label purposes. This happens when a doctor prescribes a drug generally intended for a specific type of treatment for use in treating another type of condition.

Doctors consider the practice of issuing off-label prescriptions as generally acceptable within the medical profession.

Even the Physicians' Desk Reference® or PDR, considered the medical industry's bible describing medications, notes that doctors can prescribe a specific drug for a use other than for treatments that the publication indicates for each specific medication.

For example, a doctor might decide to prescribe a certain anti-depressant drug as treatment for a sleep problem, although literature on that particular medication never specifics or indicates such a use.

Because of this "off-label" prescription process, an individual sleep-deprived patient faces a wide array of potential treatment options. What eventually gets selected often hinges largely on the particular physician, the diagnosis and perhaps even what an individual doctor prefers to prescribe for certain sleep-related medical conditions.

Consider non-addictive natural substances

For the most part, only standard allopathic physicians hold licenses enabling them to prescribe potentially addictive narcotics like benzodiazepine, non-benzodiazepines and anti-depressant medications.

By contrast, homeopathic physicians often prescribe or recommend natural and non-addictive sleep remedies considered unlikely to cause harmful side affects. However, the general public rarely hears about these various natural substances. These include Valerian Chamomiles, passion-flower, 5HTP, Kava-kava and melatonin.

That's partly because huge multi-national pharmaceutical companies produce the potentially lucrative narcotics or drugs prescribed by standard-practice allopathic physicians. These giant firms, sometimes referred to as "Big Pharma," stand to earn billions of dollars from the sale of these risky drugs.

Compounding the problem, the huge drug companies would generate little if any revenue by promoting and distributing natural substances. The law prohibits Big Pharma from patenting nature-made products, a process that would enable individual firms to corner the market on such remedies.

Worsening matters, the costs to consumers and insurance companies can reach hundreds of dollars per prescription for sleep medications produced by Big Pharma. By comparison, many natural remedies suggested by homeopaths are as little as $10 or much less.

All along, some pharmacies sell or offer the many of the nature-made substances over-the-counter, enabling consumers to make such purchases without prescriptions.

Meantime, however, Big Pharma spends perhaps hundreds of billions of dollars on TV commercials promoting sleep-related, potentially addictive drugs.

Consumers need to make tough choices

Ultimately, consumers must decide which type of sleep remedies they're more willing to risk taking and to pay for. Some choices invariably hinge in large part on advice a patient receives from a physician or other medical professional.

From the start, patients should keep in mind that a homeopath is far more likely to prescribe a non-addictive natural substance than would a standard allopathic doctor.

"Natural substances or remedies are always preferable, especially when considering that sleep occurs naturally in healthy people," said James W. Forsythe, M.D., and H.M.D., often considered among the nation's leading oncologists and homeopathic physicians.

Rather than simply running to the store and buying natural substances in hopes of curing sleep problems, anyone with such an ailment should first see a licensed physician or homeopath for a thorough examination, Forsythe said.

Medical experts use their expertise in determining the best-possible remedies, and these professionals also can determine whether a specific sleep problem stems for any of many potentially serious causes such as heart ailments.

In addition, certain natural substances require a prescription, such as injectable HGH, which rejuvenates youthful characteristics including sleep among maturing people.

Complicating matters even more, some allopathic physicians might argue that as an overall form of medicine, homeopathy fails to adequately or scientifically test various natural substances for their apparent or possible levels of effectiveness.

Herein a controversy erupts, a battle of the minds among those in the allopathic medicine community tied to Big Pharma—verses homeopathic physicians who stress the importance of considering so-called natural or nature-made remedies.

CHAPTER 19

Homeopathic sleep remedies abound

Through hundreds of years of testing within various cultures world-wide, people from diverse societies and medical practices have found and use natural substances that they say provide remedies or cures for many ailments—including certain persistent sleep problems.

Numerous natural substances also contain extremely minute quantities of potentially toxic materials. Such factors increase the importance of following the advice and recommendations of a licensed and certified homeopath.

Among substances most often recommended by homeopathic physicians or listed in published reports for sleep problems, following thorough examinations of patients:

● **Arsenicum album**: Often sold in tablet, liquid or powder form as "tinctures" for treating specific conditions such as insomnia, allergies and anxiety, homeopaths generate this substance by baking nickel, cobalt or iron at high temperatures in order to eliminate arsenic.

● **Cocculus**: Some homeopaths reportedly consider this substance, commonly called "moonseed," found primarily in warm tropical climates, as an ideal remedy for people who complain they're too tired to sleep.

● **Ignatia amara**: According to some homeopathic literature, derivatives from this pear-shaped fruit found in China and the Philippines might help people who suffer from insomnia as a result of personal trauma or extreme grief that occurs due to the loss of a loved one.

● **Lycopodium**: Sometimes called "Wolfpaw clubmoss" or a variety of other names, and once used for flash-powder in early photography and found in nature worldwide, this reportedly helps people who wonder if they have slept.

● **Nux vomica**: Derived from evergreen strychnine trees found in Southeast Asia, this might help people suffering from hangovers or substance abuse, who also experience insomnia.

● **Silicea**: Also called "silica," this comes from flint, a hard sedimentary substance, once used by Native Americans to make tools.

● **Sulphur**: Often hailed as "sulfur," this is found naturally in certain minerals, sometimes considered helpful for insomnia that results from insufficient exercise. A lengthy list of natural herbs provide sulstones, including valerian, chamomile, passion-flower, St. John's Wort, certain sleepy teas and various over-the-counter preparations.

CHAPTER 20

Many health problems inhibit sleep

While many people might immediately blame sleep problems on stress or anxiety, researchers often say a variety of other health issues sometimes ignite such difficulties.

Pain or discomfort from arthritis, heartburn, cancer or a wide variety of other ailments sometimes prevents people from sleeping throughout the night. Individual situations sometimes worsen, since the resulting lack of rest prevents healing.

This vicious or potentially deadly cycle often causes concern among physicians, who sometimes target the underlying health issue rather than concentrating on sleep difficulties. To be sure, conquering pain or discomfort often can go a long way toward putting an individual patient's regular sleep habits back on track.

"I've slept all night for the first time in weeks or even months," a patient might say, after receiving the correct amounts of specific pain medications—rather than drugs that have a primary indication for addressing sleep problems.

"Concentrate your thoughts on the work at hand," said Alexander Graham Bell, the inventor of the first practical telephone, who died in 1922 at age 75. "The sun's rays do not burn until brought to a focus."

With this need to focus in mind, physicians and sleep experts often look for a variety of possible lifestyle choices, activities or foods that might adversely impact their patients' natural abilities to sleep.

A 1996 Gallup Poll indicated 60 percent of people over age 50 report that pain awakened them on occasion. Some maturing people complained that health problems forced them to lose about two hours of sleep nightly, nearly 11 nights each month.

Compounding this problem, numerous other medical conditions or diseases that cause varying levels of pain rob people of valuable or important sleep. These conditions include fibromyalgia, neuromuscular diseases, asthma, lung problems, bronchial spasms, chronic sinusites, angina and migraine headaches.,

Sleep difficulties plague children

Rather than afflicting just middle-aged or mature people, sleep problems also can plague children—potentially hampering their concentration and their need for lengthy rest.

Some physicians, educators and parents urge children to get adequate sleep, partly in order to prevent mood problems while enabling them to concentrate. Largely for these reasons, pediatricians sometimes recommend that parents instill good, regular sleep habits in their youngsters beginning at an early age.

Preferably starting at the toddler stage, a child should prepare for bedtime by following a pre-designated and predictable routine, physicians say.

Always fashioned as a positive experience, this process might involve brushing teeth, putting on pajamas, saying prayers and hearing or listening to bedtime stories.

Meantime, parents or care givers should ensure children can sleep in a restful, comfortable environment without distractions that might awaken them. Ideally, a child's bedroom or sleeping area should remain at moderately cool or room temperatures.

Well into their teenage years, a child's bedroom should lack potential distractions such as TVs, computers or video game equipment. Keep lighting at constant, unchanged levels throughout the night.

Beginning as early as the toddler stage, children should be discouraged from needing their parents nearby in order to fall asleep. Just as important, parents or care givers should discourage all youngsters from awakening during wee hours of the night. Partly in an effort to achieve this pattern, the adult should refrain from staying with the child until he or she falls back asleep.

Controversy erupts regarding sleep time

The impacts of monthly menstruation and eventually menopause often inhibit or interrupt the abilities of individual women to get necessary sleep, scientists say.

Even so, women who sleep about seven hours a night rather than eight hours nightly might live longer, at least according to one recent study. In 2004, the National Center for Biotechnology Information reported that recent studies suggested "the risk of (death) is lower in those sleeping seven hours."

In the study conducted in cooperation with the Division of Sleep Medicine at the Department of Medicine at Boston's Brigham and Women's Hospital, women in 1986 answered a mailed questionnaire about sleep duration.

Of the 82,969 women who responded to the study initial questionnaire, 5,409 of them died in the 14-year span through the year 2000, according to the researchers' contact with relatives coupled with information provided by the National Death Index.

"Mortality was lowest among nurses reporting seven hours of sleep per night," a report on the study said. Researchers noted that women who sleep less than six hours and more than seven hours nightly "remained associated with an increased risk of death," after adjusting for such factors as history of cancer, smoking, exercise, depression and age.

"These results confirm previous findings that mortality risk in women is lowest among those sleeping six to seven hours," the report said. "Further research is needed to understand the mechanisms by which short and long sleep times can affect health."

Numerous other studies reportedly have indicated longer life spans for people of both genders who sleep 6-7 hours per night.

However, in 2002, a news report on the Cable News Network or CNN quoted some sleep experts who "immediately sought to debunk the conclusions as flawed and said they will only cause confusion."

The controversy or differences of opinion erupted as some medical professionals continued to recommend the longtime standard eight hours of nightly sleep.

The CNN report described a study published by the Archives of General Psychiatry, which "included 1.1 million men and women, and found the highest survival rate among those who sleep six to seven hours a night."

CNN said the National Sleep Foundation, which recommended

eight hours sleep per night, "immediately attacked the study's findings, and said they can do nothing but cause the public unnecessary confusion and concern."

CNN quoted an official from the Northside Hospital Sleep Medicine Institute in Atlanta as saying that "the data can't be used to establish a cause and effect relationship because there are flaws in the study."

With these disputes in mind, major questions might erupt. Among the many possible questions: How do you feel after a full night's sleep? Shouldn't we just let nature take its course?

While such disputes might persist, medical researchers seem persistent in their efforts to study sleep, while developing possible methods to maximize the many benefits from this activity.

Unique male responses during sleep

While various controversies continue to focus on the best possible duration of sleep, medical professionals acknowledge a longstanding fact—that the male penis often or invariably becomes erect during deep rapid-eye-movement or REM sleep.

On a technical level, physicians call this occurrence "nocturnal penile tumescence" or NPT. Other than individuals who suffer from varying levels of erectile dysfunction, virtually all healthy males from puberty and older experience this.

Often hailed across North American cultures as "morning glory," this condition might be considered a potential sign or indication of overall good health for an individual male.

Amazingly, however, even in the wake of major advances in overall medical technology, some physicians or biologists might insist they lack a definite reason why NPTs occur. A 2005 report in the "Journal of Endocrinology" stated that hormonal neurons in the brain stem during sleep might generate such erections.

When attempting to determine if a man's inability to achieve erection while awake is based on biology or mental attitudes, health experts study the individual's physical condition during sleep. If a man's penis becomes erect during REM, doctors might reach a diagnosis concluding that his condition is physiological in nature—rather than physiological.

Although not as noticeable, according to some medical accounts women sometimes experience clitoral erections while sleeping.

Even for scientists and well-educated physicians, all the many specific variables and unique attributes of sleep seem difficult to comprehend or to understand.

"I would rather live in a world where my life is surrounded by mystery than live in a world so small that my mind could comprehend it," said Harry Emerson Fosdick, an American clergyman who died in 1969 at age 91.

Maintain adequate temperatures

The temperature in your immediate environment while sleeping plays a key factor in determining the quality and duration of sleep. To enable this basic biological process to perform at peak efficiency, always strive to rest in areas where temperatures feel comfortable and pleasing.

This strategy might become challenging amid what some scientists call global climate change, where some regions become increasingly warm or even dangerously hot.

Extremely hot or very warm conditions fight against the body's natural tendency to sleep within temperature variations that feel extremely comfortable. Thus, if parts of the globe are heating as some scientists indicate the weather changes could adversely impact peoples' abilities to sleep during healthful conditions worldwide.

"The first wealth is health," said Ralph Waldo Emerson, the philosopher and poet. Within this realm of thinking, we must take proactive action to ensure optimal conditions for sleep. This means taking aggressive measures to help guarantee that you and your relatives or loved ones always sleep in pleasantly comfortable temperatures. Among some of the many suggested ways scientists say we should accomplish this:

● **Control temperatures**: Partly in order minimize energy costs, close windows and shades during hot daylight hours to keep at least some cool temperatures inside your living area. And during warm-weather periods, open windows at night to allow cool air inside.

● **Drink fluids**: Drink plenty of fluids since excessive heat might cause you to perspire profusely during sleep, a condition that potentially could result in serious health problems.

● **Air conditioning**: Those who can afford air conditioning should consider purchasing and installing such systems, especially in regions that become extremely hot during summer.

● **Motor homes**: Extremely dangerous or deadly conditions can emerge in stationary motor homes when inhabitants run air conditioners. So, use caution if living in such a dwelling.

- **Sleep outside**: A lack of air conditioning and excessive heat might force many people to sleep outside. Anyone faced with this predicament should consider building cool temporary tent-like shelters, while using repellants to hinder insects.

- **Social environment**: Especially during extreme emergencies caused by seriously high temperatures, some communities might open neighborhood shelters in schools or public buildings. Consider staying at such facilities if and when other options fall through.

- **Humidity**: Depending on their personal preferences, some individuals might feel more comfortable when using humidifiers or even when placing ice in front of cooling fans.

- **Common sense**: Always remain cognizant of potential problems excessive heat might cause, potentially hindering your ability to sleep—and always remain alert or creative in seeking solutions to these various problems.

According to some weather experts, global climate change also might cause extreme decreases in temperature—at least temporarily—in some widespread regions. As a result, you also should consider taking appropriate measures to make sleep comfortable during very cold temperatures.

Just 10,000 years ago, a relatively short time frame in a geologic sense, much of North America experienced its most recent ice age. Some scientists claim similar conditions might emerge soon, especially if people continue using massive amounts of fossil fuels.

CHAPTER 21

Sleep hygiene and positioning

Which side of the body should you sleep on, to achieve optimal health?

Most people become surprised to learn that the various positions we assume while sleeping can and do affect certain aspects of our health, especially after age 50.

While seldom considered important in the young or middle ages, these sleeping hygiene hints can make a difference between high- and low-quality sleep patterns. Based on longtime research and frequent findings, experienced medical professionals recommend these positions to lessen or eliminate symptoms of certain specific medical conditions:

Left side: For stomach reflux or gastroesophageal disease, mature patients with snoring problems, emphysema, venous blood under low pressures, and fluid buildups in the left lung. In these instances, the three-lobed right lung is able to breathe more efficiently during sleep than the two-lobed left lung.

Right side: Sleep here if fluid has built up on the right side of the chest cavity, or if the patient suffers cardiomyopathy, referred to by lay people as a "flabby heart."

The back: Mature patients with snoring problems should avoid this position, sleeping instead on their left sides.

Hand and arm positioning: Avoid sleeping with your hands or arms above the head if you suffer arthritis or tendonitis of those appendages, or numbness or tingling of the hands, a condition sometimes associated with carpel tunnel syndrome.

In addition, people with specific medical ailments should consider certain physical sleeping aids, such as thin or very soft pillows between or under affected joints or limbs for individuals with arthritis. A rolled towel under the neck often helps people who suffer arthritis in the neck or cervical spine.

For patients with gout, or painful toes from arthritis, accidents or injuries, consider using a footboard to keep the sheets and every blanket off the affected toes.

CHAPTER 22

How much quality sleep
Do you owe yourself today?

From the perspective of some people, the process of sleep mirrors a pay-as-you-go system. Under this realm of thinking, heralded as the "sleep debt" process, a person who sleeps only a few hours daily for a week or so would essentially need to "pay back the body by catching up on the amount of sleep that has been lost."

While such strategies might seem like nonsense to many of us, some sleep experts and physicians seem to have varying opinions on the apparent validity of such claims.

Amid the ensuing debate, a 1997 report in the "Journal of Sleep Studies" chronicled a study at the University of Pennsylvania's School of Medicine, indicating an impact on the daytime sleepiness of people who have been deprived of their sleep. Various other sleep-debt studies also have been conducted, some apparently indicating a need to catch up on lost snooze time, according to various published reports and media accounts.

Hoping to reach definitive conclusions, some scientists or sleep researchers have conducted what they call sleep onset latency or SOL tests. This process attempts to measure the specific changes that occur when an individual progresses to and from wakefulness and deep levels of rapid-eye-movement sleep.

When an individual persistently and consistently experiences a need or craving to sleep, depending on specific conditions and test results, scientists or sleep experts might diagnose that person as suffering from "excessive daytime sleepiness" or EDS.

Key questions facing some researchers might involve whether a person's persistent and consistent episodes of EDS have resulted from his or her "sleep debt"—going for excessive periods without getting adequate daily sleep.

Some people might sleep too much

From the perspective of non-trained lay people, the mysterious process of sleep might seem even more perplexing when we acknowledge that some people apparently sleep too much—or at least far more than most other individuals.

Sure enough, in what non-experts might label as the polar opposite of excessive daytime sleepiness or instances when people sleep only a few hours daily for lengthy periods, some individuals suffer from hypersomnia.

People with this condition experience their daily sessions of nighttime sleep for prolonged periods of time. According to information published by the National Institutes of Health, in conjunction with the U.S. National Institute of Neurological Disorders and Stroke, people with hypersomnia:

● **Naps**: Often want to take repeated naps throughout the day, sometimes amid times, places or activities that society considers inappropriate. People with hypersomnia sometimes strive to go to sleep in the workplace, during conversations or while eating.

● **Wakefulness**: "Patients often have difficulty waking from a long sleep, and may feel disoriented."

● **Various symptoms**: A wide variety of other symptoms might ocur, everything from anxiety to decreased energy and a loss of appetite. Other symptoms sometimes include restlessness, memory problems, slow speech and thinking too slow.

● **Social interaction**: "Some patients lose the ability to function in family, social, occupational and other settings."

According to these reports, researchers have pinpointed a variety of possible causes that might generate hypersomnia. Besides sleep disorders like sleep apnea, disorders within the autonomic nervous system have been cited as a possible reason.

Adding to the complexity of this research, medical professionals also report that they're looking into possible outside forces such as alcohol abuse or drug abuse.

"In some cases it results from a physical problem, such as a tumor, head trauma, or injury to the central nervous system," the report says.

Vital research on the problem continues

Concerned about the impacts of hypersomnia, sleep experts continue to conduct vital and important research that many people from the general public have never known about.

For instance, undaunted and persistent in their efforts to pinpoint causes, these medical professionals have concluded that tumors, central nervous system injuries and head trauma also might cause at least some instances of hypersomnia.

"Medical conditions including multiple sclerosis, chronic fatigue syndrome, depression, encephalitis, epilepsy or obesity may contribute to the disorder," said the report issued by the National Institutes of Health.

Researchers noted that a genetic propensity toward hypersomnia might get passed to subsequent generations. Adolescents and young adults suffer from this condition more than any other age group.

Hoping to address this condition, some physicians prescribe or recommend a variety of medications, mostly expensive drugs produced by Big Pharma.

Meantime, some sleep experts steer away from recommending drugs, or suggesting lifestyle changes; instead, these medical professionals might attempt to remove daily routines that likely triggered the onset of hypersomnia in an individual. These choices might range from kicking the habit of regularly attending late-night parties to leaving graveyard-shift jobs.

Beware of microsleep problems

Microsleep, the intermittent and unpredictable episodes when a person snoozes for brief periods, hails as among the most dangerous of the many sleep disorders.

People suffering from microsleep sometimes fall asleep from one to 30 seconds, often without knowing they drifted off. Some instances involve people who suddenly realized they had been driving, without any recollection of what happened during the previous several seconds.

"As soon as there is life there is danger," said Ralph Waldo Emerson, the widely acclaimed philosopher, poet and essayist. Indeed, the mere act of living entails widespread inherent risks. Nonetheless, conditions such as microsleep push danger factors up to extremely life-threatening levels.

While the causes of microsleep reportedly might include a wide range of factors, individuals with this condition must strive to keep such occurrences at manageable levels.
Some researchers indicate they fear microsleep incidents have led to serious accidents, and that future similar catastrophes likely will occur.

According to a 2004 press release issued by Loughborough University's Sleep Research Centre in the United Kingdom, microsleeps "normally occur when people are tired but trying to stay awake." Several prescription drugs emerge as useful for this condition including Provigil® and Ritalin®.

Important: Visit your doctor

The many intricate sleep-related disorders or conditions, coupled with the basic need to snooze, make it clear that people should visit their doctors at the earliest sign of such problems. Waiting to see if a symptom or an apparent disorder "goes away on its own" could enable or provide an environment for that specific condition to worsen.

"Nip it in the bud," some seasoned medical professionals might say. Just as a cancer caught or found early in its development sometimes is easier to cure, correcting or eliminating a specific sleep condition might help prevent subsequent health problems.

With such strategies in mind, you should also remain aware that some specific sleep problems—other than the classic disorders already mentioned—might signal current or possibly future health difficulties. Among the most prevalent of these instances:

● **Exploding head syndrome**: Within a few hours after falling asleep, people with this condition believe they hear extremely loud noises within their heads. While some researchers cite stress or anxiety as possible causes, seizures have been mentioned as possible causes.

● **False awakening**: People suffering from this condition sometimes experience dreams, mental stories in which they seem to awaken—but in reality the individual remains fast asleep. For some individuals, this illusion emerges as so convincing that they honestly believe they had awakened.

● **Hypnagogia**: Within this mysterious state between snoozing and wakefulness, an individual might experience difficulties or interesting perceptions when drifting into or out of sleep.

● **Hypnic jerk**: While beginning to fall asleep, a person involuntarily twitches—so severely in some instances the individual might even appear as if startled. Scientists and researchers reportedly have a variety of theories on the causes, possibly related to slowdowns in muscles, breathing and heartbeats as bodily functions transition into the sleep phase.

● **Drowsiness**: Sometimes called "somnolence" by physicians, this condition emerges when the person feels a strong motivation to fall asleep. Just like microsleep, this condition can pose serious danger when the person attempts to engage in everyday activities such as driving.

James W. Forsythe, M.D., H.M.D

Intriguing sleep facts can become fun!!

While the many various sleep disorders and resulting complications might seem daunting, discovering various other intriguing facts about snoozing can generate intrigue and even a sense of fun or intrigue. Learning these details can provide compelling topics to liven up your party conversations, possibly sparking curiosity in others.

"The public have an insatiable curiosity to know everything, except what is worth knowing," said Oscar Wilde, the Irish playwright and author.

Many people dislike know-it-all characters who strive to seem far more intelligent or worldly than anyone else. Anyone learning these enticing details can keep the info to themselves, or share as much information as they want. Among some of the most intriguing or puzzling behaviors that sleeping can generate:

Bed bugs

As children, while preparing for bed or after getting tucked in for the night, many of us heard our parents or care givers lovingly proclaim: "Don't let the bed bugs bite!"

For the most part, many children seem to give such rhymes little thought, perhaps since most youngsters never learn that such tiny creatures exist. These miniscule nocturnal insects sometimes feast on the blood of various warm-blooded hosts—often people.

These little bloodsuckers, classified by scientists within the cimicidae family of insects, enjoy living in the same areas as human beings. As a result, bed bugs enjoy swarming to the same types of environments where people enjoy sleeping—including between the covers and sheets of beds.

Many people mistakenly believe bed bugs never grow large enough for us to see them. However, wingless and reddish-brown while in the adult stage, these oval and flattened creatures are large enough for the naked human eye to observe. In fact, bed bugs often grow up to five millimeters in length.

People unlucky enough to sleep with bed bugs might discover to their great displeasure that these insects prefer to begin eating about one hour before dawn—but can attempt to feed at any time throughout the day.

According to some published reports, bed bugs can go for lengthy periods of time without feeding, perhaps many months. Yet when ideal opportunities arise, these creatures might choose to feast at least every five days to 10 days or so.

Amazingly, many people fail to realize that quiet and undetected bed bug infestations may enjoy consistently feeding on them over a period of time. Scientists warn that these pests, which can feast anywhere on the surface of your body, often feast while the victim or host remains unaware of these feedings.

All along, some people might mistakenly guess that filthy environments or unwashed human flesh attracts these insects. To the contrary, bed bugs become attracted to the warmth of a person coupled with the carbon dioxide that the individual exhales.

According to some published accounts, many people believed that insecticides caused a widespread eradication of bed bugs across the

United States through the mid- to late-1900s. But various news reports indicate a resurgence nationwide, as the overall problem persists worldwide.

Knowing this, have you ever experienced tiny red bumps or welts on your body? If so, these might be the result of bed bugs that feasted on your blood, quite possibly while you slept. Intense itching sometimes erupts on the surface of the body where bed bugs have eaten, apparently the result of saliva that bed bugs insert into the blood of their victims.

Perhaps understandably, some people who learn or discover that bed bugs have been feasting upon them become stressed or anxious, sometimes suffering insomnia.

Understandably, anyone who suspects he or she has been bitten by bed bugs should take some or all of the following measures:

• **Physician**: Visit a certified physician or medical professional, preferably as soon as possible. Only a doctor or experts in such matters can diagnose such a condition, and prescribe appropriate medicines.

• **Pest control**: Consider seeking the help of licensed, qualified and experienced pest control companies. While eradicating such insects might sound easy, removing or exterminating these pests can become an intricate process.

• **Washing**: Some people might want to wash their bedding or sheets, followed by processing in clothes dryers where temperatures exceed 120 degrees Fahrenheit, at least according to various published reports.

- **Other hosts**: While some people believe that bed bugs prefer human blood, scientists say these insects also will feast on other warm-blooded mammals such as mice or even common pets such as cats or dogs. People who suspect or find bed bug infestations in their homes should consider bringing their pets to a veterinarian for a checkup.

In summary, bed bugs and the problems they cause emerge as no laughing matter, particularly among people who become shocked at discovering such instances. Luckily, though, we can minimize these hassles by taking a limited number of precautions, or basic steps after finding such events have occurred.

Power Naps

Some people like taking brief power naps, in an effort to eliminate or prevent sleepy situations.

People who employ such strategies strive to awaken from power naps before the eventual onset of rapid-eye-movement or REM-sleep and slow-wave sleep. If or when those sleep stages commenced, the power-napper would have to awaken during a regular or normal phase of snoozing in order to complete pre-scheduled activities.

According to some medical literature, when people awakened too soon from the normal deep phase of sleep they often feel groggy or disoriented, suffering from a condition called "sleep inertia." Marked by declines in the person's ability to move in a normal, coordinated fashion, such grogginess could last up to three hours when the individual gets disturbed during daytime hours.

With these negative potential outcomes in mind, some power-nap practitioners strive to limit such snoozes to 20-minute periods.

176

A 2005 report on NASA's official government Web site said astronauts sometimes take naps at specified times, rather than face potential irritability, forgetfulness and fatigue after they previously fail to get adequate sleep.

"The bottom line—we should stop feeling guilty about taking that 'power nap' at work or catching those extra winks the night before our piano recital," said a 2002 report and press release issued by the National Institutes of Health.

The Institutes' declaration on the importance of power naps noted that a study at Harvard University showed that sleep and naps "appear to enhance information processing and learning." According to the report, the Harvard experiments showed that a "midday snooze reverses information overload and that a 20 percent overnight improvement in learning a motor skill is largely traceable to a late stage of sleep that some early risers might be missing."

College students have discovered that learning retention improves after power naps due to a process called "retroactive inhibition." This process allows for more learning retention after a mind-clearing nap.

In additional measures unrelated to the focus of this study, some people take "caffeine naps"—which entail power-naps followed by ingesting caffeine-laden drinks or pills in an effort to increase alertness.

Chronotype

Various studies have consistently shown that individual people give differing answering when asked at which times of the day they feel most alert.

Some people indicate they awaken early, before experiencing their most alert and energetic periods during the first portion of a day. By contrast, other groups of individuals feel far more alert during the latter half of the day and stay up late at night.

This situation gets more complex when certain individuals within each category take these natural preferences to what some observers might consider an extreme—staying up extremely late each night or awakening many hours before sunrise each morning.

All along, while a vast majority of individuals indicate at least some preference to either alertness during mornings or evenings, many refrain from leaning toward either extreme, at least according to some researchers.

On an even more specific basis, some scientists apparently believe that "morning people" generally share certain lifestyle preferences such as eating, sleeping and activity habits—while "evening people" supposedly share their own general propensities.

Sleep and creativity

Some people believe that sleep, coupled with the dreams that snoozing makes possible, generates a condition that enables an individual to become creative or to develop ideas.

Paradoxically, still other individuals embrace the notion that perhaps insomnia does just as much or more to inspire or energize the creative mind.

"Problems cannot be solved by the same level of thinking that created them," Einstein said.

According to a 1964 news report in the "San Francisco Chronicle," golf great Jack Nicklaus—considered one of history's all-time greatest professional golfers—told a reporter that he had a dream that enabled him to improve his golf swing.

"I tried it the way I did in my dream and it worked," the Chronicle quoted Nicholas as saying. "I shot a 68 yesterday and a 65 today ... I feel kind of foolish admitting it, but it really happened in a dream."

A 1988 article in the "Journal of Sleep Research and Sleep Medicine" describe a study indicating that people lose creativity when deprived of sleep. And a 2004 article in "Nature" chronicled a study indicating that people who get eight hours of nightly sleep displayed a greater ability to develop insights into specific tasks, when compared to people deprived of adequate snooze time.

The same year, CBS News reported that there "may be new meaning to the phrase 'sleep on it.'" The news story told of a "Nature" article about a study by German scientists, suggesting that getting eight hours of sleep at night can stimulate creative thinking the next day."

Sleep and learning

Some researchers believe sleep plays a key function in our ability to remember information and to learn.

A 2004 article in "Nature," entitled "Sleep Inspires Insight," described research indicating that sleep sometimes can give a person a quick insight into integral information or knowledge.

Also in 2004, the Society for Neuroscience published a story noting that "sleep helps secure memories and aids at least some types of learning. The findings indicate that sleep is much more important than commonly believed."

Even so, the same report indicated that at least one third of people responding to a survey indicated that they get less than seven hours of sleep per night. Despite an inclination by many in the public to avoid shut-eye, findings from sleep research are leading toward better ways to:

• **Benefit**: Use sleep to "boost learning in healthy individuals and possibly those recovering from brain injuries."

• **Focus**: Increase our "respect for sleep and its ability to benefit the brain."

• **Insights**: Develop a "better understanding of how sleep and wakefulness contribute to learning."

"In particular it (sleep) seems to secure memories, termed procedural memories, which help people learn skills," the report said. "Thanks to procedural memories, you can master a video game, a gymnastics move or a melody on a piano."

CHAPTER 23

Shooting down myths about sleep

With headquarters in Washington, D.C., the National Sleep Foundation serves a valuable public service, in shooting down various myths, wives tales or misconceptions about sleep. Among the most frequent misconceptions that this organization works to discount:

• **Teenagers**: Some people mistakenly believe that any teen who sleeps during the day exhibits lazy behavior. However, teenagers need to sleep each night an average 8.5 to 9.25 hours, compared to 7-9 hours nightly for adults. The biological clocks of teenagers "also keeps them awake later in the evening and keep them sleeping later in the morning," foundation literature says. "However, many schools begin classes early in the morning when the teenager's body wants to be asleep. As a result, many teens come to school too sleepy to learn, through no fault of their own."

• **Insomnia**: Another mistaken belief leads people to think that the only problem with insomnia involves a difficulty falling asleep. However, the foundation says the other problems entail waking too early before being unable to fall back asleep, feeling unrested after awakening, and awakening often during the night.

• **Sleepiness**: Numerous people incorrectly think or assume that a person who becomes sleepy during the day must be getting insufficient sleep at night. However, the foundation says that some instances can occur even after sufficient nighttime sleep, possibly "a sign of underlying medical conditions or sleep disorder."

• **Age**: Another common misconception leads some people to incorrectly believe that "the older you get, the fewer hours of sleep you need," the foundation says. However, "while sleep patterns change as we age, the amount of sleep we need generally does not. Older people may wake more frequently through the night and may actually get less nighttime sleep, but their sleep need is no less than younger adults."

● **Reaction**: Still another belief mistakenly mandates that a person who awakens during wee hours of the morning or the middle of the night, should stay in the same position in bed and wait to fall back asleep—even if doing so involves tossing and turning or pretending to count sheep. However, "waking up in the middle of the night and not being able to go back to sleep is a symptom of insomnia," foundation literature says. "Relaxing images or thoughts may help to induce sleep more than counting sheep, which some researchers suggest may be more distracting than relaxing."

Whichever technique you use, the foundation says, "most experts agree that if you do not fall back asleep within 15-20 minutes, you should get out of bed, go to another room and engage in a relaxing activity such as listening to music or reading. Return to bed when you feel sleepy. Avoid watching the clock."

Of course, whenever sleep gets disrupted—especially on a regular or consistent basis—you should see a doctor or sleep expert to determine if an underlying biological or mental condition might emerge as a likely cause. Early signs of serious depression can include awakening too early, or an inability to return to restful sleep due to anxiety or worry.

CHAPTER 24

Quick! Take a fun and restful vacation now!

Some people might argue or insist that an average individual gets adequate rest or sleep within the home environment, eliminating the potential need for an out-of-town getaway.

Statements such as "home is where the heart is," and "you can get plenty of relaxation right where you live now," often fail to ease the minds of those who instinctively crave a much-needed trip. Perhaps the mind would "rest" or feel at ease, without having to see the same things and the same old environment day in and day out.

Travel agencies tell us that many getaways stem from a pure and simple need or desire to become tourists, to go sightseeing and enjoy recreation activities.

Even so, lots of us instinctively know or have learned through experience that leaving town can at least on occasion enable us to escape persistent everyday hassles and responsibilities—sometimes away from bothersome phones and even computer connections.

Some young adults enjoy spring breaks away from college environments, or even lengthy multi-month intercontinental excursions after graduation. Hopefully before the anticipated advent of everyday adult responsibilities, such excursions might help make the overall life experience seem well-rounded or as if the heart has gone full circle.

People much more mature in age might crave away-from-home exploration, partly as if a reward for their many years of hard and sometimes difficult work before retirement.

Whatever the inspiration for a vacation, keep in mind that such getaways might help provide excellent opportunities for rejuvenating rest and quiet time. Slow-paced activities, in turn, could re-energize the body and soul, bringing us a new zestful spirit for our returns to school, work, home responsibilities or the regular routines of retirement life.

Dedicate yourself to planning a vacation

"I need a vacation," a middle-aged husband mumbles to himself and to his wife, just about every time they drive to the grocery store every week. "We need to get out of here for awhile, to take a break but we never seem to do it. How long has it been?"

Feeling equally exhausted, the wife often echoes her spouse with similar statements: "Honey, I was just thinking the same thing. Life is far too short for us to get stuck in a rut like this. We need to get out of town."

Does such a conversation sound familiar to you, no matter what your age or economic lot in life? And do you feel better, during and immediately after those rare or frequent times when you've managed to take an out-of-town vacation by yourself or with a loved one?

Even folks who feel frustrated about the need to take a vacation should simply "just do it," perhaps if only on a limited-time, low-fund scale if financial resources are too low.

As we already know, each year many Americans skip or refrain from using all possible vacation time accrued or earned at the workplace.

However, any person who cares about himself or herself should make and carry out a focused, well-planned effort to enjoy every amount of vacation time possible. After all, don't you deserve sufficient rest time after all your hard work? Do you feel better or more enriched upon your return from getaways?

Also, if you're the family's primary breadwinner, perhaps your spouse, lover or immediately relatives could use a slow, restful, easy-going excursion as well. In many cases, you might need to take a leadership role to make that happen for them.

In order to make all this occur, focus on completing the following steps, careful to avoid skipping necessary details:

● **Location**: Either choose the destination yourself, or discuss possible locations with your mate to avoid potential confusion or misunderstandings about what everyone wants. In cases where everyone involved yearns for differing destinations, consider a compromise where one person's choice takes precedence this time—followed by the other site on a subsequent trip. In the process, refrain from instigating unnecessary conflict.

● **Activities**: Where potentially strenuous always-on-the-go activities emerge as the focus of many vacations, take deep thought beforehand on planning for "slow" activities or on finding an environment conducive to rest. Also, once you arrive at a destination, perhaps some people within a family or group can choose to enjoy lots of activities, while others might enjoy their preference of essentially staying put "at the home base."

● **Budgeting**: Some financial planners urge clients to avoid taking too many vacations, since money spent on such getaways potentially could accumulate over the years—perhaps in some instances over a period of years growing to levels sufficient enough to augment retirement incomes. Yet as a general rule, many people might proclaim "balderdash to that," since life needs to have at least some balance.

● **Staycations**: A play on the word "vacations," and sometimes referred to as "stay-cations," these so-called excursions essentially entail staying at home during a vacation period rather than traveling—perhaps for financial reasons. Those who choose this option might decide beforehand to eliminate potential distractions from the home environment. To do this, consider unplugging the telephone or stashing cell phones, and avoiding email or other potential quickie forms of mass communication.

● **Frequency**: Rather than taking a single one-month-long yearly vacation, some people might prefer to enjoy four separate one-week vacations at regular intervals throughout the year. This way, you would always have something to look forward to, perhaps maintaining a fairly predictable mode of expected down-time from everyday stressful activities.

Leave your stress at home

Many people insist that the process of traveling in today's hectic world can generate perhaps even more stress than they already must undergo in the home environment and the workplace.

Certainly waiting in hours-long lines at airports for required security checks can tend to lead to frazzled tempers, resulting in everything from anger to exhaustion. Coupled with the inherent problems involved in jet-lag, some travelers discover that they're "dead tired" by the time they reach a destination—especially after long international flights.

To at least some of these people, going through such hassles might make the mere effort of traveling seem like too much trouble in the first place.

"Taking one lousy vacation just isn't worth all this headaches," some potential travelers might complain, also citing mega-high plane ticket costs and exorbitantly expensive airport meal expenses. While keeping all these variables in mind, you might want to try to put all these many inconveniences into perspective. Among considerations:

● **Long-term benefit**: Perhaps you're en route to a four-week stay at a quiet, secluded luxury resort, or at least to a destination considered peaceful and tranquil. Under such a scenario, perhaps you could consider the traveling phase "the brief pain before the gain."

● **Attitude**: Motivational experts tell us that a positive attitude can go a long way toward putting us in an ideal frame of mind, thereby enabling us to position ourselves for the possibility of achieving our goals. Only through such efforts can we overcome negativity.

● **Experience**: Use your own experience at traveling as a guide, or seek the advice from others with the know-how to overcome potential obstacles imposed by traveling. Read as much as possible beforehand about beneficial travel tips, or directly seek the advice of a seasoned travel expert.

● **Focus**: Once again, remember that your goal should remain to get away from home for valued rest in a unique environment. Rather than concentrating on the "hassle of the moment," consider the so-called big picture, the glorious fact that you're finally on vacation.

● **Weekend getaways**: Even three- or four-day weekend getaways can generate plenty of rest or a sense of well-being, occasionally making you feel as if the excursion lasted up to a full week. Different experiences in new environments can enable the mind to focus on important things in life, sometimes enabling us to at least temporarily forget the mundane.

Appreciate the benefits
That a vacation can provide

The mere act of driving out of town or hopping a flight to a mysterious location can jumpstart the senses, potentially generating deep sleep once we reach the destination.

Such a rejuvenating process can magnetize the brain, perhaps putting our bodies and minds in a mode capable of doing great things on the spur of the moment.

One true-life heroic story of this magnitude happened early in this century when four married women from a Western U.S. city took a one-hour trip out of town for a planned three-day getaway. Once these ladies reached their destination, a home that one of the women owned, the four of them enjoyed an evening meal and chatted late into the night—all of them drinking wine.

The next morning, they slept in, everyone getting much-needed rest before a nourishing breakfast. Later, during the late-morning hours, the host suggested that she and the other women take a brisk walk through a nearby golf course. There, the women could enjoy a blanket of fresh snow that had fallen the previous night.
Once everyone bundled up in warm clothing, the women set out

together at a leisurely pace. Blessed with an energetic and bubbly personality, Kris, the host walked ahead of the other three—accompanied by two of her beloved dogs.

Briefly out of sight from her friends, Kris watched in horror as her golden retrievers slid down a steep embankment from the golf course into an icy river. Frantic, the woman hollered for help from her companions.

Soon afterward her friends arrived on the scene. By then Kris had accidentally slid down the embankment, splashing into the icy and potentially deadly river. Afraid and yet somehow appearing quite calm, Kris struggled to get her dogs out of the river before concentrating on herself. With all her might, Kris tried to climb out of the river and up the embankment, but to no avail—her limbs flailing to and fro in the icy water.

Unless something dramatic happened right away, almost certain death would have occurred for the woman and for her pets as well.

Rest and sleep might have worked wonders

Seemingly without thinking, never taking a moment to plan, the three women outside of the water immediately took decisive action.

Determined to rescue their host and her dogs, the trio instantly formed a human chain—holding each other super-tight in order to position themselves to get this necessary job done. One woman, Patty, stood at the top of the embankment—standing firm in one place, using more of her own body strength that she ever recalled using before.

Patty held onto Linda, who braced herself halfway down the embankment in order to hold onto the third rescuer. Held by the power and determination of Patty and Linda, Kathleen braced herself at the edge of the river.

From there, Kathleen pulled Kris and her two dogs from the icy water, rescuing them from the brink of almost-certain death.

"If just one of us had let go, we all could have died," Patty proclaimed later. "This truly was a story of sisterhood, of women bonding together for a common purpose."

Were all these heroics made possible, at least in part, by the megapower of rest—the lengthy sleep that each of these women had taken the night before? Would these middle-aged women have been able to perform this combined fete, without the rejuvenating power and fulfillment that sleep can provide?

Researchers may never know for sure. Even so, some details of this tale remain indisputable, primarily that the rescuers went into action without having to plan their every move. Medical professionals say those are the types of quick reactions that sleep can enable us to instinctively perform.

Such queries, in turn, might lead us to ask additional questions as well, perhaps just as important. Could the rescuers have successfully pulled Kris from the water, if they had individually slept only a few hours the previous night? Under such a scenario, would their reaction times have been too slow to reach their friend in time?

Ultimately, the women managed to return Kris back to her home, where she promptly took a warm shower and then got plenty of rest to recuperate from the shock of her near death experience.

CHAPTER 25

Strive for a balance between
work and life

Businesses or organizations such as the Work Life Balance Centre, based in the United Kingdom, strive to enable people to control their job responsibilities—clearing the way for the possibility of these individuals enriching and enjoying their home lives.

Some sociologists believe that modern advances in technology have directly or indirectly enabled today's corporate employers to increase demands on their front-line workers. This situation, in turn, might tend to increase stress or anxiety, potentially robbing individual workers of much-needed and necessary sleep and rest time.

Many labor unions and labor organizations seem to fear that this evolutionary cycle in our economic and home environments could disrupt the necessary harmony or balance between our work and home lives.

In Madeleine Bunting's book, "Work Slaves ~ How the overwork culture is ruining our lives," the public statistics show that the time an average American spent working in 1997 reached just more than 47 hours—up more than 3 _ hours from just 20 years earlier.

According to some surveys, many people believe that advances in technology and a globalized economy have ultimately forced them to work excessive work hours.

"Living in a constant chase after grain compels people to expand their spirits to the point of exhaustion," said Frederich Nietzsche, the German philosopher and philologist.

By some accounts, the modern workplace here in the 21st Century has emerged as the single greatest stress-giver, resulting at least partly in a sharp increase in work-related disability claims. Huge responsibilities imposed by many employers require a majority of employees to continually re-educate themselves, merely in order to keep pace with never-ending technological advancements.

Recent news report indicate that just to make ends meet, in order to survive and generate enough incomes to live, some people barely have enough time to sleep. The many struggles and commitments imposed on today's workers also rob some parents of valuable quality time with their children and families.

Stung by potentially mind-boggling changes in technology, coupled with society's rapidly evolving expectations of employees, individually and collectively we all need to strive to ensure adequate time and environments for sleep to occur.

Avoid expressing satisfaction
Unless life entails more work

To their credit, many American workers seem to voice a sensible opinion that a high-quality life should encompass far more than working a 70-hour week—a situation that, sadly, seems headed for "the norm" within the requirements of corporate America.

Those eternal lyrics to the classic hit tune, "Take this job and shove it," could or should very well become rewritten to proclaim: "Take this bed and sleep here."

Pushed to the brink, past the point that common sense tells us that we should be required to work in order to achieve, some people voluntarily choose to down-size their lifestyles. Such individuals prefer to enjoy living in conditions where rest and sleep play just as big and as important of a role as exercise, education and enjoying new activities.

"Twenty years from now you will be more disappointed by the things that you didn't do than by the ones you did do," said Mark Twain, the legendary American author and humorist. "So throw off the bowlines. Sail away from the safe harbor. Catch the trade winds in your sails. Explore. Dream. Discover."

Those who embrace such a philosophy eagerly escape the boundaries imposed by corporate America. Such people find themselves willing to acknowledge and to accommodate the basic and necessary biological need and craving that we all possess for regenerative sleep and rest.

Herein let us strive to insist that as individuals, as families, as communities and as businesses, we must continue to hold a responsibility to ourselves and to the people we work with—always helping to ensure an environment or an opportunity for necessary repose.

CHAPTER 26

Appreciate the sleep clinic
And sleep medicine industries

Medical professionals within the study or specialty of "sleep medicine" dedicate themselves to researching such activity, while developing or prescribing treatments or therapies for specific related
disorders.

Major advances in sleep medicine during the past several decades
have motivated various medical organizations to meet or coordinate
efforts. Physicians and researchers want to cooperate in developing
better or more efficient ways to address related health issues.

The American Board of Sleep Medicine has been helping to coordinate such efforts, in cooperation with various prestigious organizations including the American College of Chest Physicians, the
American Thoracic Society, and the American Academy of Sleep
Medicine, according to the "Chest Journal."

The study and practice of sleep medicine has emerged as so important that physicians and various medical organizations now classify
this practice and research as a "recognized subspecialty" within the
practice of medicine.

Needless to say, at least from the standpoint of some interested observers, this interesting and important medical subspecialty seems
to be growing at an increasingly rapid rate.

The need for sleep clinics
And for sleep research intensifies

Remember that so far, researchers reportedly have identified at least 80 sleep disorders. Could the number of such serious conditions increase as scientists learn more about vital intricacies and biological functions involved in the shut-eye process?

"Intellectual growth should commence at birth and cease only at death," Einstein said. Perhaps since they sense such urgency in matters involving sleep, researchers seem to have intensified their quest for seemingly endless, still-unresolved questions about sleep.

According to various news reports, thousands of sleep clinics have opened nationwide, while the total number of such facilities worldwide apparently remains unknown.

"Sleep disorders and medical disorders of sleep are common in today's society and have significant public health implications," says a 2007 report printed by PubMed.gov, detailing a Sleep Disorders Program at UBC Hospital at Vancouver, British Columbia, Canada.

Within the program's research, the report says, scientists reviewed "data that has linked sleep restriction to a variety of adverse physiologic and long-term health outcomes including all-cause mortality, diabetes and cardiovascular disease." Meantime, the same team of scientists reviewed data demonstrating that "therapy for obstructive sleep apnea ~ is an extremely efficient use of health care resources."

As the massive 80 million-population Baby Boom generation ages and enters its senior years, such vital research could prove essential at improving and assuring the quality of life among seniors. Meantime, the need to assist the younger generations might seem just as urgent, amid overall increases in asthma and other adverse medical problems within that age range—conditions that could adversely impact the level and quality of sleep.

Advances increase the need for communication

Amid steadily increasing advances and developments in research, physicians from a variety of specialties have shown signs that they're striving to work with increasing efficiency in medical research and treatments that involve sleep.

According to information from the U.S. National Library of Medicine and the National Institutes of Health—using a process in which physicians classify health disorders—physicians strive to list various sleep problems within three basic classifications.

Physicians and medical professionals use the "Medical Subject Headings" or MeSH indexing system when establishing their various books or classifications that involve the many various life sciences.

According to MeSH reports, physicians throughout the medical community are coordinating their efforts in order to assign specific disorders with numbered codes. In this manner, doctors hope to coordinate and fine-tune specific recommended or suggested treatments for each type of condition.

These behind-the-scenes efforts seem to have enabled physicians to make significant strides in their sleep treatment efforts. And, hopefully these collective efforts will become even more efficient, especially if stress factors increase the propensity of sleep problems.

Significant advances in treatment seem likely

Let's hope that with persistence, sleep researchers will continue efforts to generate effective sleep treatments at generally low cost.

All along, a fear might persist that perhaps Big Pharma could play too large a role in mandating specific unnecessary high-cost treatments. Backed by the many billions of dollars they earn annually, the largest pharmaceutical companies have significant influence on the federal Food and Drug Administration and on standard allopathic physicians.

Within the realm of regulating which drugs to prescribe and when and how that occurs, the potential for serious problems or abuses arises. This possible predicament seems especially complex, when considering that lobbyists backed by major pharmaceutical companies carry a huge influence in Congress—which considers or develops vital legislation regulating the drug industry.

As documented earlier, many high-cost sleep drugs including highly addictive barbiturates could cause long-term health difficulties for people with sleep disorders.

Meantime, the pharmaceutical industry employs or contracts with many thousands of political lobbyists. These professionals and many of the Big Pharma companies that employ them contribute significant funds to political campaign funds, often to the same congress members who ultimately must regulate them.

With these potentially negative factors in mind, urgent and timely questions emerge. Who will look out for the so called "little guy," to help ensure that average citizens that suffer sleep problems can avoid potentially addictive drugs? How, if at all, will the FDA be encouraged to study or recommend the use of natural substances as effective treatments when possible?

CHAPTER 27

The public needs to take a pro-active role

Faced with the urgent need to help ensure good-health standards, the general public including standard physicians, homeopaths and sleep experts needs to take a pro-active role in urging cohesive and sensible treatment regulations—in conjunction with any current government administration.

To help ensure the best possible results in this regard, the public and physicians should take aggressive action in working with our government's elected leaders and with the various regulatory agencies. Among primary recommendations:

● **Health reform**: As the U.S. government continues efforts at health reform, work with Congress and the secretary of the U.S. Health and Human Services Department to ensure that sleep research and experts within this subspecialty hold a high priority.

● **Drugs**: Require the FDA to review and recommend natural substances as treatments for sleep problems, rather than solely drugs developed by Big Pharma.

● **Research**: As the health reform process gets fine-tuned, dedicate federal funds to assist research or to provide major tax incentives for those who perform such activities.

● **Lobbyists**: Restrict the seemingly unfettered access that Big Pharma lobbyists have to congress members, and limit or prohibit large pharmaceutical companies or their representatives from contributing to political campaign funds.

- **Acknowledge**: Despite any controversies that might arise, the general public and our elected leaders also need to acknowledge that in certain instances pharmaceutical products might serve as the best or most-recommended treatment methods available.

Largely in an effort to make sleep-related drugs available to U.S. citizens who truly need such medications, our nation also needs to open up the international markets to allow for the importation of such substances—but only if officials manage to implement a cost effective system designed to guarantee quality standards are met.

For consumers everywhere, the need and quality of good, nourishing and life-giving sleep remains too precious to risk at the hands of greedy companies or selfish politicians who might neglect the basic needs of society.

CHAPTER 28

Cherish the gift of sleep

Beginning in the womb till the day we die, good and sound sleep often emerges as a comforting process for the body, mind and soul as well.

To understand and to appreciate these needs is to awaken in full bloom, growing in spirit and in knowledge as we become increasingly enlightened and educated.

At any given moment throughout the remaining course of the human experience, people always will be sleeping somewhere here on earth. From the very young and innocent to the very old and dying, we all need and crave this easy and relatively free activity.

Once at rest, within the deepest phases of rapid-eye-moment, Mother Nature covers and graces us with unrequited peace. Barring any unpleasant dreams, that tranquil solitude that we first began experiencing as children can continue unabated well into adulthood.

Seemingly ensconced, perhaps at times far from the common worries imposed by the many stresses of everyday life, while at sleep our hearts and minds can open as if flowers at sunrise—perennially hopeful and eager for energy that each new day might provide.

"Life is a gift," some people like to say. And embracing and coveting such generous presents as provided by biology, let us all celebrate in the new-found knowledge that we have learned much about the blessings of sleep.

With still more advances likely regarding sleep in the near future, we can and should take comfort in the knowledge that time and time again, right up until the day we die, we can sleep and then sleep once again—enjoying our much-needed dreams and our rest as well.

Sleep

About the Author

James W. Forsythe, M.D, H.M.D.

James W. Forsythe, M.D., H.M.D., has long been considered one of the most respected physicians in the United States, particularly for his treatment of cancer and the legal use of human growth hormones. In the early 1960s, Dr. Forsythe earned his M.D. from the University of California, San Francisco, before spending two years residency in Pathology at Tripler Army Hospital in Honolulu. After a tour of Vietnam, he returned to San Francisco and completed an internal medicine residency and an oncology fellowship.

Today in Reno, Nevada, Dr. Forsythe maintains a conventional medical clinic, the Cancer Screening and Treatment Center, and a homeopathic practice, Century Wellness Clinic. A former associate professor of medicine at the University of Nevada School of Medicine, Dr. Forsythe has conducted numerous original clinical outcome-based studies on many natural substances.

For more than 20 years, he has been interested in integrating alternative and conventional medicine.

About the Editor

Wayne Rollan Melton

A former Editor-on-Loan to "USA Today," and an experienced book manuscript ghostwriter, Wayne Rollan Melton has been an entertainment columnist, society columnist and features writer, focusing in part on human behavior issues.

Other books by

James W. Forsythe, M.D., H.M.D.

"Your Secret to the Fountain of Youth ~ What they Don't Want You To Know About HGH Human Growth Hormone" (With co-author Earlene Forsythe, R.N., M.S.N., A.P.N.)

Co-Authored or Featured

Suzanne Somers' number one best sellers:
"KNOCKOUT, interviews with Doctors who are Curing Cancer" and "BREAKTHROUGH, EIGHT STEPS TO WELLNESS"

"An Alternative Medicine Definitive Guide to Cancer"

"The Ultimate Guide To Natural Health, Quick Reference A-Z Directory of Natural Remedies for Diseases and Ailments"

"Outsmart Your Cancer: Alternative Non-Toxic Treatments That Work and Alternative Medicine"

"Guide 2 Women's Health Series"

Author's request

:

Have you had a positive or negative experience regarding sleep, after reading this book? As the author prepares for follow-up publications, please visit his Website: **DrForsythe.com**

www.ingramcontent.com/pod-product-compliance
Lightning Source LLC
Chambersburg PA
CBHW060847280326
41934CB00007B/952